# DERMATOLOGY

## An illustrated guide

by

### LIONEL FRY

B.SC, MD, FRCP

Consultant Dermatologist,
St Mary's Hospital, London.

With 506 illustrations
in full colour

1978
UPDATE BOOKS

Published by
**UPDATE PUBLICATIONS LTD**


*Available in the United Kingdom and Eire from*

Update Publications Ltd
33/34 Alfred Place
London WC1E 7DP
England

*Available outside the United Kingdom from*

Update Publishing International, Inc.
2337 Lemoine Avenue
Fort Lee, New Jersey 07024
U.S.A.




*First published 1973*
*Second edition 1978*

ISBN 0 906141 02 8

Printed in Great Britain by Cox and Wyman Ltd,
Fakenham, Norfolk

# Contents

# Preface

IN the second edition of this book the basic approach to the teaching of dermatology remains the same as in the previous edition. However, a second edition has become necessary because, although diseases alter little, the approach to and management of them changes rapidly. Many treatments which were common practice five years ago are no longer used, either because adverse effects have become apparent or because newer and more effective treatments have been found. The aim of this book is not only to aid diagnosis but also to be helpful to practising doctors in their management of skin disorders.

The number of colour illustrations has been increased from 420 in the first edition to 506 in the second. This is intended to emphasize the commoner skin problems and not to show the more exotic and rare dermatoses. There is little point in presenting a dermatology textbook to the non-specialist without colour illustrations, and likewise a collection of colour illustrations without a text is not sufficient for either student or doctor. The problem of teaching dermatology is that the student cannot over a limited period of time be given a wide enough experience to be able to recognize even common lesions without difficulty, and this is the basis of the lack of confidence with which some doctors afterwards face dermatological problems.

However, the existence of colour pictures, like the opportunity to see a large number of patients, does not imply neglect of the basic approach in making the clinical diagnosis, namely, taking a good history. I have found that when students are asked to give a case presentation of a patient with a dermatological disorder they omit the history and immediately describe the rash with numerous Latin and Greek adjectives which have very little relevance to establishing the diagnosis. However, once a full and adequate history has been obtained, diagnosis can usually be confirmed by what is seen. In this book therefore, the text is designed to help the reader to an understanding of the natural history of the various conditions and how they present.

I am grateful to the following for lending me slides and allowing me to use them in this book: Dr Phillip Rodin, Dr Arnold Levene, Dr R. R. Davies, Dr C. W. Marsden, Dr C. D. Calnan and the Institute of Dermatology, Prof. K. W. Walton, Counsellor–Specialist Guidance in Public Relations and Marketing, Mr Gerald Haffenden, Dr P. P. Seah, The Leprosy Study Centre, and the Wellcome Museum of Medical Science. I also thank Photo-Optix (London) Limited for advice and help with regard to photography. I am grateful to the following general practitioners for allowing me to take photographs of acute dermatological problems not always seen in a hospital clinic: Dr John Fry, Dr J. S. Zidel and Dr J. B. Dillane.

I am indebted to the staff of Update Publications Limited, particularly Dr Kate Hope, Dr William Jackson, Mr John Snow and Mr Alan Savill, for their help with this book.

Lionel Fry

# 1. History and Examination

Even in this age of medical technology the definitive diagnosis of dermatological disorders is still made in the majority of cases on clinical grounds alone. In disorders of other systems the clinical diagnosis can be confirmed by measurement and the answer expressed in mathematical terms and the limits of normality are known. In dermatology one has to rely on a visual impression; even if the lesion is biopsied and histopathology used as an aid, one still relies on visual impressions and not definitive mathematical limits.

## History

Before beginning the examination of the skin an adequate history should be taken. Particular attention should be paid to the duration and extent of the lesions, whether they are persistent or intermittent, and if there is irritation. It is important to enquire into the past medical history, particularly for skin disease, and into the family history (one often gains a clue to the diagnosis of scabies if other members of the household are known to have similar symptoms). The occupation of the patient is important, and enquiry should be made about specific exposure to irritants or allergens.

As in disorders of other systems one should enquire about any recent stressful situations. Although it is all too common for skin disorders to be attributed to 'nerves', in some diseases stressful conditions are a contributory factor in susceptible individuals.

No history of skin disorder is complete without determining what treatment the patient has already had for the condition, and what systemic medication he may be taking for any other complaint. The former is important because the potent topical steroids (the supposed panacea for all skin disease) can alter the appearance of a bacterial or fungal infection so that it may well be misdiagnosed. Secondly, patients develop sensitivity to topical antibiotics (which are frequently added to the steroid preparations), or even to the 'bases' of the topical preparations and this perpetuates or exacerbates the original condition.

Eruptions caused by systemic medication are not uncommon and the rashes can be bizarre in their appearance leading to difficulty in diagnosis. Direct questioning about drug taking is necessary, for patients do not consider aspirin, laxatives, slimming pills, cough mixtures, etc. as drugs and do not therefore admit to taking any drugs. Patients also mistakenly believe that if they have taken drugs for a considerable length of time they cannot be responsible for a skin rash which has only been present for a short while, and they do not volunteer the required information.

## Examination

As the diagnosis in dermatology is made visually it is important to make sure the lighting is adequate.

### Type of Lesion

*Macule.* This is a flat circumscribed discoloration of the skin. If it is larger than several centimetres it may be referred to as a patch (Figure 1.1). A macule may be red (alteration in blood supply) or brown due to a pigment (melanin or haeomosiderin). Examples of this type of macule are freckles, flat moles or 'staining' following purpura.

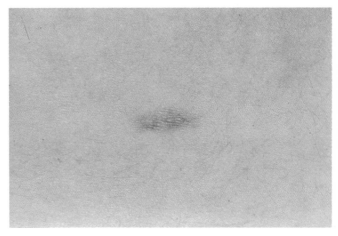

**Figure 1.1** *Macular lesion. Flat pigmented naevus.*

**Figure 1.2** *Papule. Acquired haemangioma (Campbell de Morgan spot).*

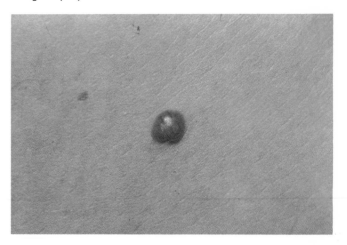

*Papule* (Figure 1.2). This is a discrete lesion raised above the skin surface and arbitrarily classified as being less than one centimetre in diameter. The majority of warts are papules.

*Nodule* (Figure 1.3). This is a raised discrete lesion measuring more than one centimetre in diameter. It is also sometimes taken to mean a lesion deeper and firmer than a papule.

*Blister*. This is a discrete collection of free fluid in the skin. If it is small, e.g. 2–3 mm, it is usually referred to as a vesicle (Figure 1.4) and if larger it is termed a bulla (Figure 1.5). Although there are specific diseases, e.g. pemphigus, dermatitis herpetiformis, which are sometimes termed the bullous dermatoses, it should be remembered that blisters are commonly seen in acute eczemas (particularly pompholyx eczema), in common viral diseases—herpes simplex (Figure 1.4) and herpes zoster, fungus infections of the feet and erythema multiforme (Figure 1.5).

*Pustule* (Figure 1.6). This is a skin elevation containing pus.

*Scaling and crusted lesions*. Scaling represents abnormality of the uppermost layer of the skin, the stratum corneum (horny layer or keratin). There may be abnormality in the formation of the keratin or it may not be shed in a normal manner. Certain types of scaling are characteristic, e.g. the white scales of psoriasis (Figure 1.7), the yellowish scaling of seborrhoeic eczema or the brown scaling of some forms of ichthyosis (Figure 1.8).

*Crusts* are the dried remains of serum, which may occur in an acute inflammatory condition, such as acute eczema or impetigo, and have a yellow colour (Figure 1.9).

## Distribution of Lesions

Considerable help in arriving at the correct diagnosis can be gained from the distribution of the lesion; certain common diseases show predilection for certain sites, e.g. psoriasis—elbows, knees, sacrum and behind the ears; atopic eczema—flexures of the limbs; acne—face and upper trunk; pityriasis rosea—the trunk with the long axis of the oval lesions along the lines of cleavage; scabies—wrists, between the fingers, genitalia in males and breasts in women; erythema nodosum—extensor surface of the legs (and occasionally arms).

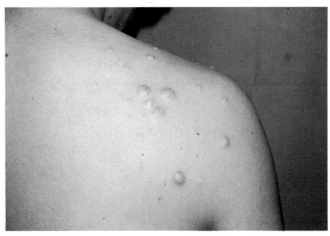

**Figure 1.3** *Nodules. Neurofibromata.*

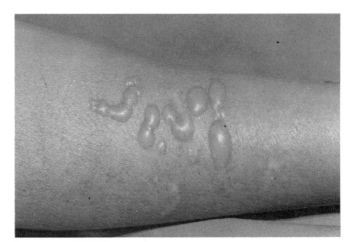

**Figure 1.5** *Large blisters (bullae) in erythema multiforme.*

**Figure 1.4** *Small blisters (vesicles) in herpes simplex.*

**Figure 1.6** *Pustule in acne.*

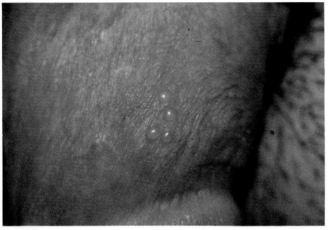

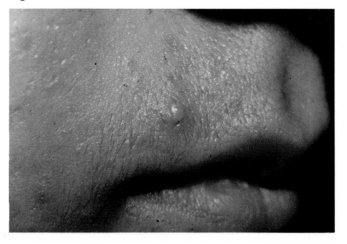

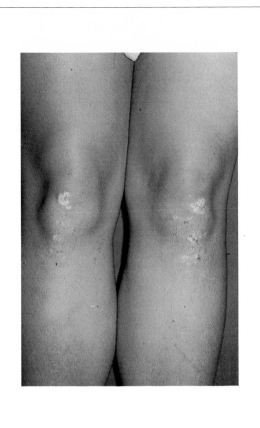

**Figure 1.7** *White scaling of psoriasis.*

**Figure 1.8** *Brown scaling found in some forms of ichthyosis.*

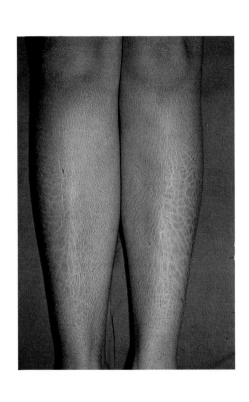

## Configuration

Certain patterns may be suggestive of a diagnosis, although none is absolutely diagnostic:

*Linear.* Lesions of this type, particularly in lines of trauma (Koebner phenomenon), occur in viral warts, psoriasis and lichen planus (Figure 1.10). Some naevi are also linear.

*Annular.* Fungal infections are the best known annular lesions (e.g. ringworm, Figure 1.11), but it is a common mistake to diagnose all annular lesions as fungus infections. Partially treated or clearing psoriasis often has an annular pattern (Figure 1.12). Urticaria, pityriasis rosea and a condition of unknown aetiology called annular erythema can all be represented by annular lesions.

*Grouped lesions.* Grouped blisters are characteristic of herpes simplex, herpes zoster and dermatitis herpetiformis, and grouped papules are commonly found in molluscum contagiosum (Figure 1.13).

*Symmetry and asymmetry.* Disorders due to external factors such as viruses (Figure 1.14), bacteria, and fungi (Figure 1.15) tend to give rise to asymmetrical eruptions. Diseases

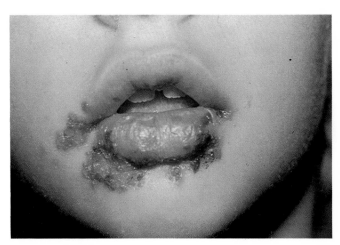

**Figure 1.9** *Crusts in impetigo.*

**Figure 1.10** *Linear lesion. Koebner phenomenon in lichen planus.*

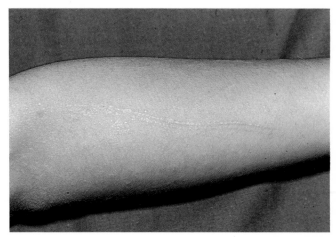

3

**Figure 1.13** (Right) *Grouped papules in molluscum contagiosum.*

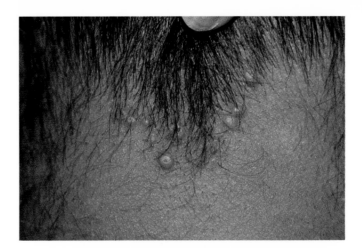

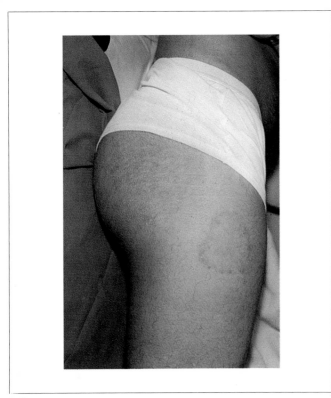

**Figure 1.11** *Annular lesion in fungal (ringworm) infection.*

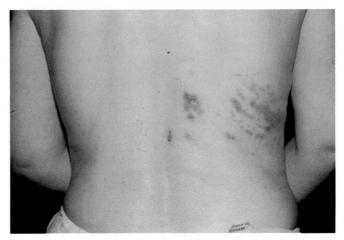

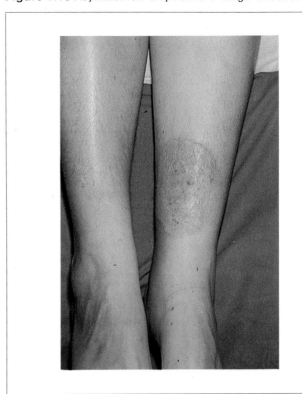

**Figure 1.14** *Asymmetrical eruption in herpes zoster.*

**Figure 1.12** *Annular lesions in resolving psoriasis.*

**Figure 1.15** *Asymmetrical eruption in a fungal infection.*

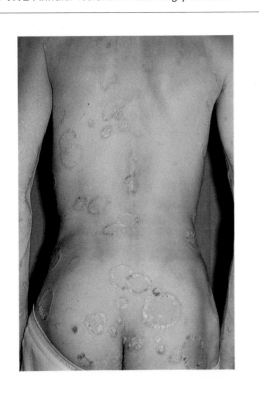

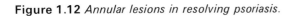

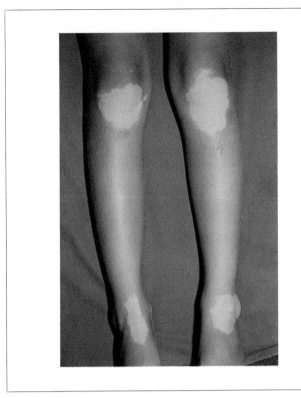

**Figure 1.16** *Symmetrical lesions in vitiligo.*

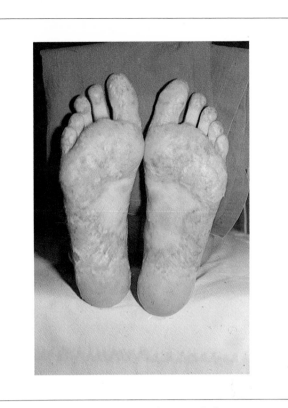

**Figure 1.17** *Symmetrical lesions in pompholyx eczema.*

**Figure 1.18** *Symmetrical lesions in atopic eczema.*

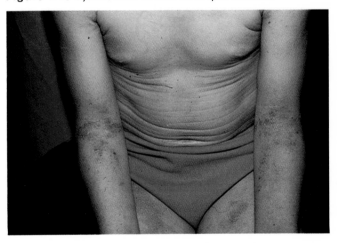

due to internal factors, so-called endogenous disorders, e.g. lichen planus, vitiligo (Figure 1.16) and the 'internal' eczemas (Figures 1.17 and 1.18) usually give rise to symmetrical eruptions.

### Additional Points

It is often well worthwhile examining the buccal mucosa and nails either for confirmatory evidence or a clue to the disease. For example, in lichen planus there is often involvement of the buccal mucosa as evidenced by white streaks or patches (Chapter 9), and small pits (like pin-pricks) are often found in the nails in psoriasis (Chapter 8).

# 2. Eczema: Clinical Features and Classification

THE terms 'eczema' and 'dermatitis' tend to be used synonymously, eczema being commoner this side of the Atlantic and dermatitis in the United States. Eczema is derived from the Greek word *ekzein* meaning to boil over or break out, and in this book eczema will be used in preference to dermatitis.

### Definition

Eczema denotes a special sequence of inflammatory changes in the skin, which, though similar, can vary from patient to patient. Likewise the clinical features can vary depending on the severity and/or chronicity of the disease and the site involved. The principal signs are redness (Figure 2.1), swelling (papules or oedema), blisters (large or small, Figure 2.2), scaling which may be loose and thin (Figure 2.1), or thick (hyperkeratosis, Figure 2.3) depending on how the normal process of keratinisation is affected; exudation of serum, which may be severe leading to weeping, or moderate and mix with the scales of the skin to form crusts (Figure 2.4). Fissures or splits (Figure 2.5) may occur particularly on the palms or soles. Thickening of the skin referred to as lichenification (Figures 2.6 and 2.7) is particularly likely to occur as a result of continued scratch-

ing in atopic eczema. Changes in pigmentation may occur, and this may be seen as hyper-pigmentation (Figure 2.8) or hypo-pigmentation (Figure 2.9). This physical sign is most apparent in coloured people and is sometimes the most obvious sign of the eczema. Purpura or bleeding into the skin is not common but may occur after continual scratching, particularly on the legs.

The appearance of any particular case of eczema may include one, two or several of the above features, and thus one case of eczema may vary from another. In addition, the eczema in an individual patient may vary from one site of the body to another, e.g. an acute weeping eczema on the hands, with spread of the eczema to the forearms and trunk, appearing there as an erythematous papular eruption.

It should be emphasised that the changes occurring in the skin in eczema are completely reversible, and it is often helpful for the physician to be able to stress this point when the patient consults him.

### Classification

The classification of eczema is difficult and not very satisfactory. This is because in the past some of the terms used to describe eczema have been based on the appearances of

**Figure 2.1** *Erythema and scaling in subacute eczema.*

**Figure 2.2** *Small blisters in acute eczema.*

**Figure 2.3** *Hyperkeratotic scaling in chronic eczema of the hands.*

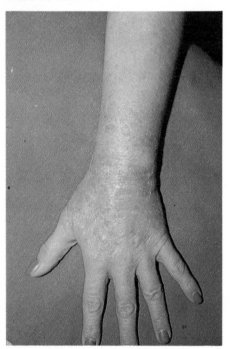

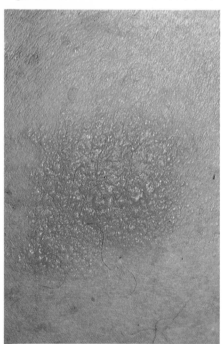

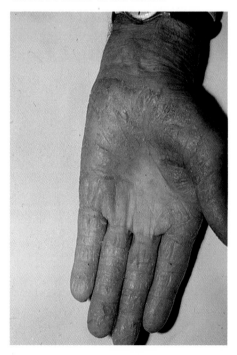

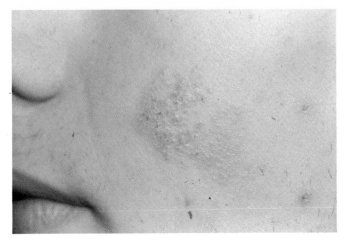

**Figure 2.4** *Yellow crusts in subacute eczema.*

the eruption, while others have been based on so-called aetiological factors, or specific sites of the eruption. Thus there has been considerable overlap in the terminology, one type of eczema having three or four names depending upon which criteria are used.

At the present time the eczemas are divided into two main groups; first, that in which the eczema is due to specific *exogenous* factors, and second, that in which there are no specific exogenous factors, the eczema sometimes being termed *endogenous*. This subdivision is important because if there are exogenous factors they must be identified, for if they can be avoided this in itself may result in a cure.

Unfortunately exogenous eczema does not have a specific morphological pattern but shows the same features which may be exhibited by an endogenous eczema. However the distribution of the eczema (Figure 2.10), the occupation of the patient, and direct questioning concerning self-medication with topical preparations and cosmetics etc. may well give a clue to whether or not the eczema is due to exogenous factors. In some instances, such as eczema caused by metal earrings (Figure 2.11), lipstick, or an article of clothing, the distribution and localisation of the eczema suggests the diagnosis. But eczema due to a constituent of an ointment, either the drug itself or the base (Figure 2.12), may be extremely difficult to diagnose unless one is aware of the possibility as there are no specific sites and it is often super-imposed on an endogenous eczema to which the patient has been applying the ointment.

Exogenous eczema is usually subdivided into (a) *true allergic or immunological* eczema, in which the patient has an allergy to a certain substance, (b) *irritant or toxic* eczema in which the substance damages the skin directly and in which there is no immunological reaction.

The classification of endogenous eczema is more difficult because it is not based on any scientific principle but on gross morphological appearances and the sites of the body that may be affected. Confusion often arises because more than one term is used to describe one particular type of eczema, e.g. atopic, infantile, flexural; or the blistering eczema that occurs on the palms and soles is referred to as dyshidrotic eczema, pompholyx or discoid eczema. Until we understand more about endogenous eczema the classi-

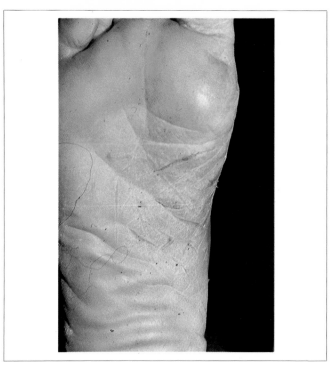

**Figure 2.5** *Fissures (splits) in chronic eczema on the sole.*

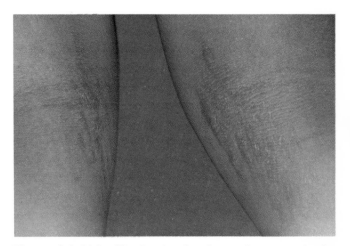

**Figure 2.6** *Lichenification in chronic atopic eczema in the antecubital fossae.*

**Figure 2.7** *Lichenified patch of eczema on the leg (lichen simplex).*

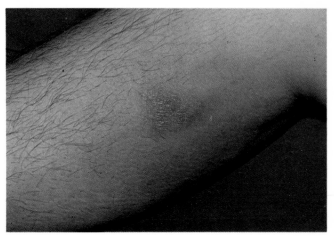

7

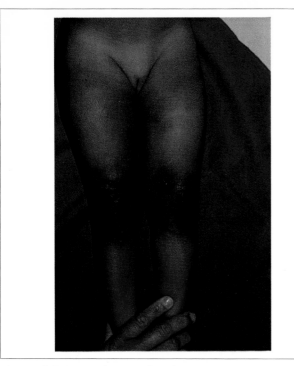

**Figure 2.8** *Hyperpigmentation due to eczema.*

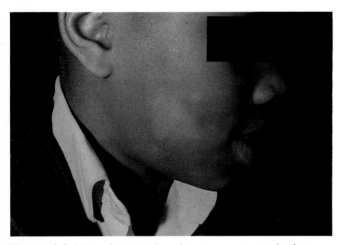

**Figure 2.9** *Hypopigmentation due to eczema on the face.*

**Figure 2.10** *Localised eczema on the back of the thighs due to sensitivity to an antiseptic applied to a lavatory seat.*

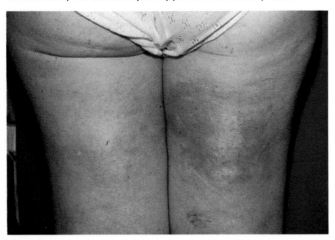

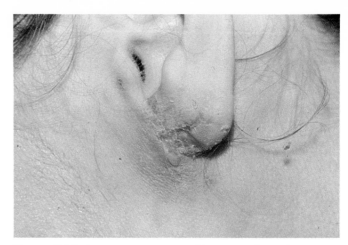

**Figure 2.11** *Acute eczema caused by a metal ear-ring.*

fication will have to remain arbitrary based on clinical criteria as follows.

1. *Atopic eczema*. This is the commonest type of eczema seen in childhood, and is often associated with a family history of asthma and hay-fever.

2. *Seborrhoeic eczema*. This derives its name from the fact that the sites involved are those with the greatest sebum production per area of skin surface, e.g. scalp, face, back and chest.

3. *Nummular or discoid eczema*. This derives its name from the clinical appearances, i.e. it occurs as small circumscribed areas of eczema.

4. *Varicose or hypostatic eczema*. This is eczema which occurs on the lower leg and is associated with impaired venous drainage of the limb.

5. *Pompholyx eczema of the hands and feet*. This tends to be symmetrical occurring on the palms and soles, the sides of the digits and their dorsal surface over the distal two phalanges.

It should be emphasised that this classification may not be complete enough to cover all the endogenous patterns of eczema encountered, but it will serve as a useful guide for further discussion. It should also be stressed that eczema often does not occur in the clearly defined patterns found in any descriptive classification. Any type of eczema (endogenous or exogenous) may lead to spread of the eruption, so-called autosensitisation (Figure 2.13), with more general involvement of the skin, which if it becomes complete is referred to as *erythroderma* or *exfoliative dermatitis* (Figure 2.14).

Table 1. Classification of eczema

| Exogenous | Endogenous |
|---|---|
| Primary irritant | Atopic |
| Allergic | Seborrhoeic |
| (Antigen-antibody reaction) | Nummular or Discoid |
| | Varicose |
| | Pompholyx or Hand and foot |

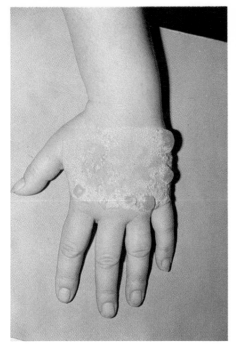

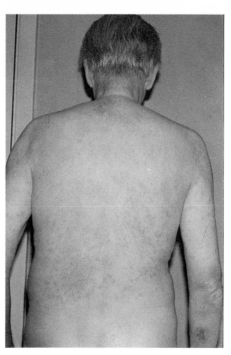

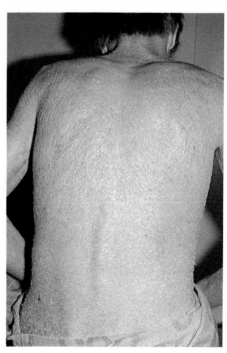

**Figure 2.12** *Acute blistering eruption caused by idoxuridine lotion applied to the hand in the treatment of herpes simplex.*

**Figure 2.13** *Widespread eczema on the arms and trunk due to pompholyx eczema on the hands.*

**Figure 2.14** *Exfoliative dermatitis (erythroderma).*

# 3. Exogenous Eczema

ECZEMAS in this group are caused by the skin coming into contact with chemicals, natural or synthetic. There are certain clues which may be present and should be looked for in establishing a diagnosis of exogenous eczema. In the early stages a sharp delineation between the affected skin and the normal skin may be apparent (Figure 3.1). Some sites are more commonly affected than others and there are three factors which determine these sites. First, certain parts of the body are more likely to be in contact with chemicals e.g. hands, face, neck and genitalia (by transference of the chemicals from the hands). Second, the thickness of the skin varies—if the hands are exposed to chemicals, the eruption is more likely to appear first on the back of the hands then on the palms, because the skin is thinner on the back and the chemicals are more easily absorbed (Figure 3.2). Third, the absorption of chemicals into the skin is enhanced by moisture and thus parts of the body which secrete larger amounts of sweat, or where the evaporation of sweat is impaired by opposing skin surface and lack of air (e.g. groins, axillae and flexures of the limbs) are more likely to be affected. This point is well illustrated by contact eczema due to stockings in which the eruption first appears on the feet and popliteal fossae due to greater absorption of the allergen into the skin at these sites. Contact eczema has also to be considered when the distribution of the eruption is localised to one particular area and is asymmetrical (Figure 3.3).

### Spread

The eruption in contact eczema ranges from a faint erythema to an acute blistering. It should always be borne in mind that eczema may subsequently appear at other sites of the body which have not been directly in contact with the chemical. This spread of the eczema may be due to 'autosensitisation' from the primary eczematous skin or due to absorption of the exogenous chemicals which affect the skin at distant sites (Figure 3.4). Although this secondary spread of eczema may affect any part of the skin, it has a tendency to spread to certain sites with some allergens. For example, eczema due to nickel sensitivity frequently spreads to the skin around the eyes and ante-cubital fossae (Figure 3.5). This may be the pattern presenting to the physician and the patient may not mention her 'suspender rash' which she may have had for years. At present the factors which cause eczema to spread to secondary sites are not fully understood but some eczemas spread after a matter of days and others only after months or even years, with continuing eczema at the primary site.

### Cause

The cause of contact eczema may be a primary irritant (non-allergic) or an allergenic (sensitising) agent.

### Primary Irritant Eczema

Substances which cause this type of eczema may be divided into two classes.

#### Strong

These are usually caustic substances with which patients

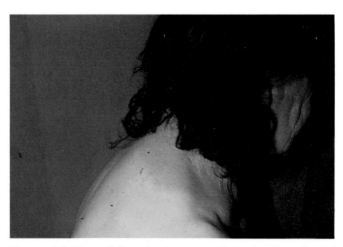

**Figure 3.1** *Sharp delineation between affected and unaffected skin in contact eczema caused by hair dye.*

**Figure 3.2** *Contact eczema caused by chromium salts in cement. The eruption is at this stage on the back of the hands but not the palms because of greater absorption of the allergen through the thinner skin on the back of the hand.*

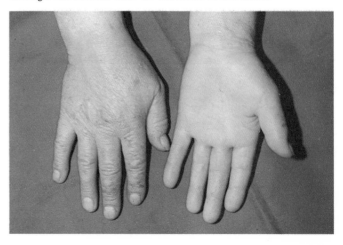

### Blisters

Only the large blisters need to be pricked as these increase irritation and general discomfort.

### Systemic Therapy

*Corticosteroids.* These are required, and justifiable, only in a small number of patients with contact eczema in whom the eruption is very extensive and acute. The commencing dose should be approximately 30 mg prednisone daily, and this should be reduced by amounts of 5 mg daily as soon as the condition begins to improve.

*Antibiotics.* Not infrequently acute eczema becomes secondarily infected. The infecting organism is most commonly a staphylococcus and/or a streptococcus, and an appropriate systemic antibiotic should be given. If there is no response within one or two days, a swab should be taken for culture and sensitivity. If the eczema becomes impetiginised (i.e. a superficial bacterial infection occurs) then topical antibiotics in an appropriate base are also helpful. The antibiotic of choice is probably fusidic acid because of the low incidence of resistance of staphylococci and streptococci to this antibiotic. Ideally swabs should be taken for culture and sensitivity.

*Antihistamines and sedatives.* An acute eczema is very irritating and causes a great deal of discomfort. Oral antihistamines such as promethazine 25–50 mg at night or trimeprazine 10 mg two or three times a day are helpful because of their anti-pruritic and hypnotic action. If the patient is agitated, diazepam 5 mg t.d.s. is helpful.

# 4. Atopic Eczema

Eczema in infancy is most commonly atopic and thus the term *infantile eczema* is used by some authorities synonymously with atopic eczema. It is also referred to as *flexural eczema* as the flexor aspects of the limbs are among the commonest sites to be affected. It should, however, be remembered that atopic eczema can occur in adults, and involve any part of the skin, so 'atopic' is used in preference to 'infantile' and 'flexural' to describe this form of eczema.

The term 'atopic' was originally used to mean 'strange' but because this type of eczema is associated with asthma and/or hay fever, the name was subsequently used to imply 'allergic' eczema. Atopen has been used in the past to mean allergen or antibody. However, at the present time atopic eczema is not thought to be due to any exogenous allergens. The exact cause of this type of eczema is unknown, but it is now considered to be one of the endogenous forms of eczema.

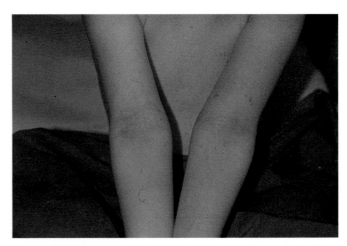

**Figure 4.2** *Atopic eczema in the antecubital fossae.*

**Figure 4.3** *Involvement of the face in atopic eczema.*

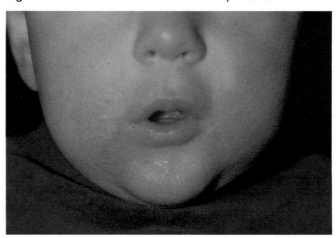

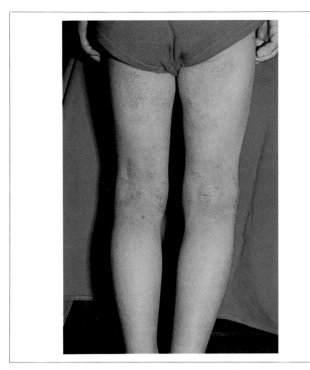

**Figure 4.1** *Atopic eczema in the popliteal fossae and on the back of the thighs.*

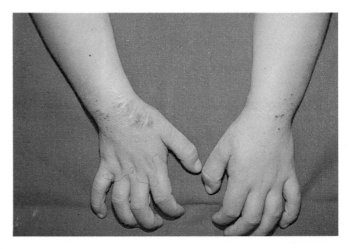

**Figure 4.4** (Right) *The hands and wrists are common sites of involvement in atopic eczema.*

16

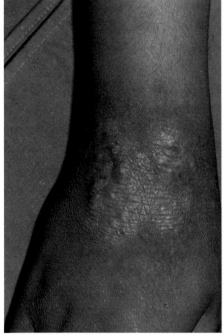 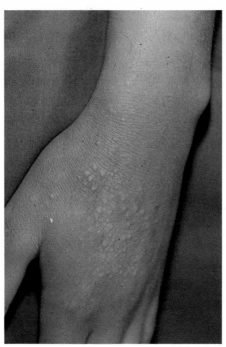 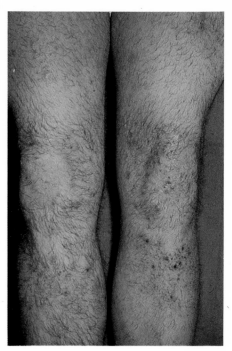

**Figure 4.5** *Thickening or lichenification of the skin caused by continual scratching in atopic eczema.*

**Figure 4.6** *Papular form of lichenification.*

**Figure 4.7** *Excoriated atopic eczema.*

### Age Incidence

Atopic eczema is not present at birth and usually does not occur before the age of three months. The commonest time, of onset is during the first and second years of life, although it may present for the first time later in childhood.

### Distribution

The most .frequent sites are the popliteal fossa (Figure 4.1) and the antecubital fossa (Figure 4.2), but face (Figure 4.3), neck, wrists and hands (Figure 4.4) are also commonly involved. This eruption is usually symmetrical, and if a unilateral or a solitary lesion presents then alternative diagnoses must be considered. Occasionally the eczema may spread from the usual sites and large areas of the skin become affected, particularly the arms and legs. Very rarely does the condition become generalised.

### Type of Lesion

The typical physical signs to be seen are erythema, scaling and thickening of the skin (lichenification, Figures 4.5 and 4.6). The features of acute eczema, i.e. crusting and weeping are not common but may occur; blisters are very rare. Atopic eczema is a very irritating condition and excoriations with bleeding are frequently seen (Figures 4.7 and 4.8). Lichenification is thought to be a response of the skin to continual scratching.

Alteration in pigmentation of the skin, either hypo- or hyper-pigmentation (Figure 4.9) may occur, particularly in coloured children where there may also be small (1–2 mm) fine papules on the trunk in addition to the more typical lesions described above.

Because of the excoriations and since, as in most skin disorders, the protective function of the skin is lost, secon-dary bacterial infection is not uncommon, and this may present as pustules or purulent crusted areas.

A physical sign sometimes seen in atopic eczema is white dermographism. If the red eczematous skin is firmly stroked with a blunt instrument, a white line appears a few moments later (Figure 4.10).

### Natural History

Atopic eczema is a very common disorder and the results of various surveys have shown that between one per cent and ten per cent of the population may be expected to have some degree of atopic eczema during childhood. In the majority of those affected the eczema is very mild and will probably clear permanently before the child is five. This type of eczema is subject to exacerbations, and the child may be clear for many months in between flare-ups. The causes of the exacerbations are not usually obvious, but climatic and emotional factors can sometimes be incriminated. Atopic eczema is usually better in a climate which is warm but of low humidity and is aggravated by cold and wind. The eczema is frequently made worse by emotional problems and stressful situations.

In the vast majority of children, perhaps 95 per cent, the eczema will clear permanently in childhood, but in a small number it will persist into adult life. It is not possible to give the parents an exact age when the condition will resolve because of subsequent outbreaks which may occur even after months or years and this should always be mentioned at the first interview.

### Family History and Associated Conditions

Atopic eczema is associated with asthma and hay-fever. The three disorders together are referred to as the atopic

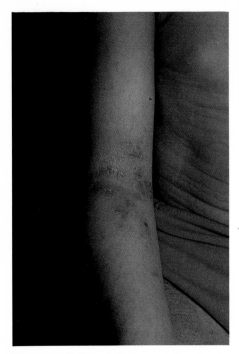

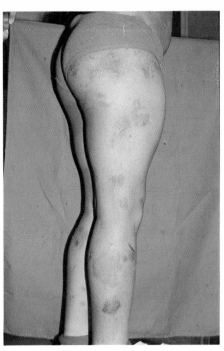

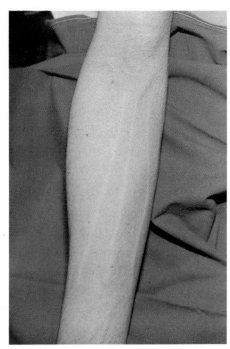

**Figure 4.8** *Excoriations and fissures in subacute atopic eczema.*

**Figure 4.9** *Post-inflammatory hyperpigmentation in a negro child with atopic eczema.*

**Figure 4.10** *White dermographism in atopic eczema.*

syndrome, but it should be stressed that the majority of atopic subjects will only develop one of the three disorders. The atopic syndrome is genetically conferred and there is frequently a positive family history of one of the three complaints when a child with atopic eczema is seen for the first time. The exact mode of inheritance is as yet unknown but it seems to be a dominant trait.

Only a small number of patients with atopic eczema will develop asthma or hay-fever in later life, probably as teenagers or in early adult life, and by then the eczema has usually cleared.

### Management and Treatment

Once the diagnosis of atopic eczema has been made it is very important to explain the natural history of the complaint to the parents. Unless this is done they will be disappointed and will tend to lose confidence in their doctor each time there is a flare-up or reappearance of the eczema.

*Topical treatment.* Atopic eczema being, like other eczemas, an inflammatory condition of the skin, the basis of treatment is the counteraction of inflammation with anti-inflammatory substances.

In the *acute* phases when there may be weeping or oozing, drying lotions and compresses are indicated. For the hands and feet potassium permanganate at a strength of 1:8,000 made up in warm water is suitable. Physiological saline is an effective alternative and it has the advantage of not staining the skin brown. One per cent hydrocortisone lotion or cream should be applied after the soaks or compresses and the area covered with clean linen.

In the commonest form of atopic eczema the skin is red, dry and scaly. The basis of treatment is topical

corticosteroid preparations. However, it must be stressed to the parents (and patients if old enough) that topical corticosteroids are not 'curative' but suppressive, and will control the eczema if used correctly. There are three important points to note in the prescribing of topical corticosteroids in the management of atopic eczema. First, and most important, is the strength of the steroid used. It must be appreciated that the potency of topical steroids varies from that of one per cent hydrocortisone to that of clobetasol propionate which is approximately 1,000 times greater. In between there are many other topical steroids of varying potency, and it is important for the doctor to learn the strength of these topical steroids compared to one per cent hydrocortisone so that he has a full range of steroids of varying potency available for use. The reason for avoiding the use of potent topical steroids in atopic eczema is the side effects of these drugs (see Chapter 25). The important side effects are a product of the strength of the steroid and the length of time for which it is used. Thus it is permissible and justifiable to use potent topical steroids for a short duration to clear eczema. Ideally the doctor should try to keep the eczema under control with a relatively weak topical steroid, but should be prepared to use the more potent preparations for short periods, e.g. two weeks, when the eczema proves refractory. However, the intervals between courses of potent topical steroids must be carefully controlled and these drugs should not be given on 'repeat prescriptions' without seeing the patient.

The second important point is that sufficient of the topical preparation should be given to the patient, so that he does not run out of ointment after a week or so and then feel reluctant to trouble the doctor again. The quantity of preparation prescribed will therefore be proportional to the extent of the disease. If the eczema is very extensive then approximately 200 to 300 g may have to be prescribed. In this instance it may well be better and more economical to dilute stronger topical steroids rather than to prescribe the proprietary preparations in small tubes. The diluent required depends on the preparation being used and can be found in the External Diluent Directory (see Chapter 25). It seems sensible for the physician to learn the appropriate diluent for one potent topical steroid ointment and another for a cream, and then to vary the strength as required rather than to change from one steroid to another.

The final point to consider is the base of the topical steroid. If the eczema is dry and scaly then an ointment is indicated, but if the eczema is exudative a cream is more appropriate.

### Systemic Therapy

*Antihistamines.* Atopic eczema is a very irritating condition sometimes interfering with sleep and thus antihistamines such as promethazine hydrochloride and trimeprazine tartrate are helpful particularly at night time. They should be given approximately one hour before the child is due to go to bed.

*Antibiotics.* If the eczema becomes secondarily infected, antibiotics will be required. If there are only small pustules or crusting (impetiginised eczema) then topical antibiotics may be sufficient to clear the infection. However, if there is inflammation of the deeper parts of the skin and subcutaneous tissues, manifested by swelling, redness, lymphangitis and lymphadenopathy, then systemic antibiotics will be required. If the infection is severe, topical steroids should be discontinued or changed to very weak preparations only. A number of topical antibiotics, e.g. fusidic acid, neomycin and gentamicin, are combined with topical steroids in proprietary preparations.

*Systemic steroids.* By far the majority of cases of atopic eczema are controllable with topical steroids. If the disease is extensive and not responding to topical measures this may be an indication for systemic steroids, particularly in adults, but fortunately these cases are becoming extremely rare, since the advent of newer topical steroid preparations.

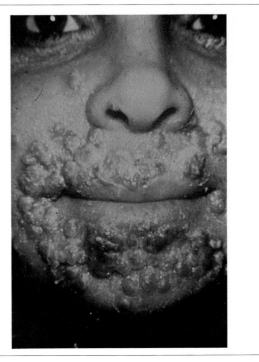

**Figure 4.11** *Kaposi's varicelliform eruption in a child with atopic eczema.*

*Immunisation.* Atopic eczema is considered a contra-indication to vaccination against smallpox because of the risk of developing a widespread secondary viral infection with vaccinia virus—known as Kaposi's varicelliform eruption. (Figure 4.11). Although this complication of vaccination is rare it does have a mortality rate of approximately 10 per cent. It should also be mentioned that a similar condition can occur in patients with atopic eczema from infection with the herpes simplex virus, and the condition is clinically indistinguishable from that caused by vaccinia virus.

There is no absolute contra-indication to immunisation against other disorders but it is best to carry these out when the eczema is in a state of remission, or very minimal.

# 5. Varicose Eczema and Ulceration

THE term varicose eczema is used synonymously with stasis or hypostatic eczema and the condition is considered to be due to venous stasis. Varicose veins may be present, but there are other causes of venous incompetence in the legs, and varicosity of the superficial veins is frequently not seen on examination of patients with this type of eczema. Incompetence in the deep veins of the legs or a previous thrombophlebitis predispose to this type of eczema.

### Site

The commonest site for varicose eczema and ulceration is the medial side of the leg just above the malleolus (Figures 5.1 and 5.2). The eczema may spread to the lateral side of the leg and/or to the dorsum of the foot and involve the whole leg (Figure 5.3). Like any other eczema the condition may affect any area of the skin and become widespread, and occasionally this is the presenting feature in varicose eczema.

### Appearances

The eczema usually first begins as a red patch which may be associated with some slight oedema of the ankle. Subsequently the area becomes scaly (Figure 5.1) and in the chronic state the scales become pigmented and have a greasy appearance. Varicose eczema is often purpuric and in the chronic state the skin surrounding the eczema is often pigmented (Figure 5.1). This may be due to melanin, haemosiderin or both. Lichenification and vesiculation are usually not seen in this type of eczema.

The eczema may be persistent for many years without showing much alteration or the skin may break down and ulceration develop (Figure 5.4). Occasionally patients with no preceding eczema on the legs sustain a slight injury to the lower leg which subsequently develops into a 'varicose' or 'hypostatic' ulcer with little or no surrounding eczema. (Figures 5.5 and 5.6). In these patients there must be underlying venous stasis. Because of the chronicity of these ulcers and their poor venous drainage there is often secondary bacterial infection with crusts (Figure 5.6) and/or pus formation. However, if there is no varicose eczema of the legs it must be seriously considered whether the ulcers may be due to some underlying condition such as peripheral arterial disease, blood dyscrasias, nodular vasculitis, poly-

**Figure 5.1** *Varicose eczema on the lower medial aspect of the leg. Pigmentation is often seen and the scales have a greasy appearance.*

**Figure 5.2** *A varicose ulcer in the commonest site just above the medial malleolus.*

**Figure 5.3** *Varicose eczema which has spread to involve most of the leg.*

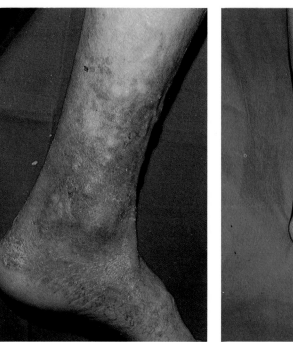

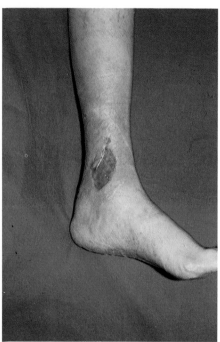

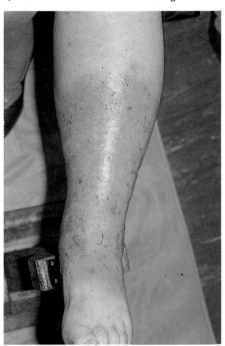

arteritis nodosa, or a manifestation of a drug eruption.

A physical sign sometimes seen in association with long-standing hypostasis is 'atrophy blanche' (Figure 5.7). The whiteness of the skin is due to atrophy and scar formation, and telangiectasia is present in this type of skin lesion.

### Treatment

Apart from the direct treatment of the eczema and ulcers, measures to counteract the hypostasis are of paramount importance.

1. *Postural drainage.* Elevation of the feet when sitting should be encouraged whenever possible. Raising the foot of the bed by approximately nine inches frequently helps to heal varicose ulcers which have otherwise proved resistant to treatment. If possible the patient should also lie on the raised bed for half an hour during the day, particularly if there is a tendency for fluid to accumulate in the lower leg.

2. *Standing.* Avoidance of prolonged periods of standing is important in the treatment and further prevention of varicose eczema and ulcers. Walking is far less harmful as the muscle activity increases venous return.

3. *Supportive stockings and bandages.* Elastic stockings should be recommended in the early stages of mild developing oedema, or when the eczema and ulcers have healed, to prevent further trouble.

In the definitive treatment of the eczema and/or ulcers more elaborate supportive measures are required. If there is no superadded infection of the ulcers and/or eczema, bandages impregnated with tar or zinc paste can be applied directly to the leg. The paste bandage is then covered with a firm elastic bandage. These bandages can be left in place for one or even two weeks. It is important that they are applied correctly and the bandaging should be carried out by the district nurse at home or in the out-patients' department. The bandages have a healing action brought about by the zinc or tar, and give support. It should be stressed that bandages must be applied from just proximal to the toes to just below the knee. If daily or even twice daily topical treatment to the ulcer or eczema is required, then paste bandages are not suitable. In these circumstances an elastocrepe is applied from the ball of the foot to just below the knee, over the dressings used in the treatment of the eczema and ulcers. If stronger support is required and can be tolerated by the patient, then a Bisgaard or blue-lined bandage should be applied.

### Topical Treatment for Eczema

In the *acute* stages the patient should rest in bed for a short time, with the leg elevated and protected by a cradle, and the eczema is treated with compresses of potassium permanganate 1:10,000. Clean linen dressings should be used at this stage. As the eczema settles and becomes sub-acute, 1 per cent hydrocortisone cream should be applied to the skin twice daily, the leg covered with tube-gauze and a firm supportive bandage, e.g. elastocrepe. In the later stages more powerful topical steroid preparations are sometimes helpful but these should be used with caution, for if ulceration develops the steroids will delay healing and often enlarge the ulcer. It is wise to dilute the proprietary preparations approximately 10 times in a suitable cream base. The cream is applied once or twice a day and covered with tube-gauze and a supportive bandage. Alternatively in the chronic forms of varicose eczema even without ulceration, one may use either the occlusive tar or zinc paste bandages as described above.

**Figure 5.4** *Chronic varicose eczema associated with ulceration.*

**Figure 5.5** *Extensive varicose ulcer with normal surrounding skin.*

**Figure 5.6** *Infected varicose ulcer.*

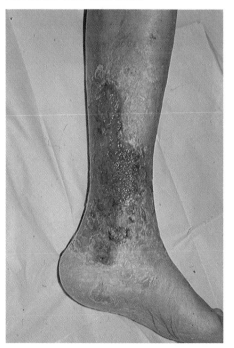

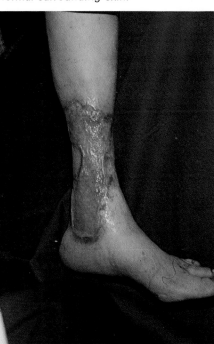

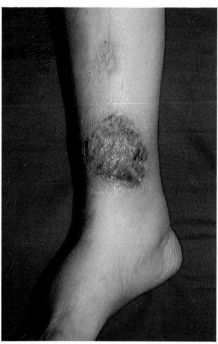

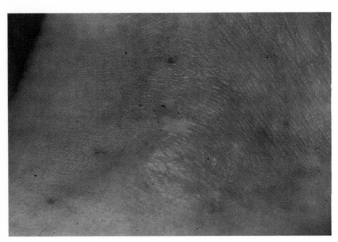

**Figure 5.7** *'Atrophy blanche'. Scarring of the skin which is occasionally found in association with varicose eczema and/or ulceration.*

**Figure 5.8** *Exacerbation of eczema surrounding an ulcer due to sensitivity to an ointment preservative.*

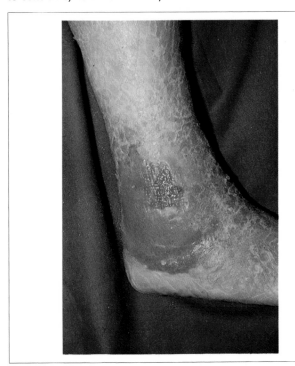

## Topical Measures for Ulcers

Most varicose ulcers seen for the first time are secondarily infected. A swab should be taken for culture and the ulcer cleaned with a solution of equal parts of eusol and paraffin. If there is a considerable amount of debris and pus the ulcer should be cleaned twice a day. The ulcer should be covered with a non-adhesive dressing followed by an elastocrepe or blue-lined bandage. To increase the chances of healing it is helpful to apply pressure to the ulcer with a sorbo rubber pad over the dressing and bandaging over the pad. If it is not possible to clear the infection of a varicose ulcer by the above measures, then antibiotics may be required. These should be used after a swab has been taken for culture and sensitivity of the organisms. Antibiotics may be used systemically or topically. However, it must be stressed that there is a high incidence of patients with varicose eczema and/or ulcers becoming allergic to topical antibiotics, particularly neomycin and soframycin. This may in part be due to the chronicity of the condition, causing the antibiotics to be used for a long time, or it may be due to altered skin structure associated with varicose eczema. Once the ulcer is clean and not infected, and the patient is ambulant, then occlusive paste bandages are helpful in the management. The bandages may be applied as described above, and need only be changed at weekly or two-weekly intervals.

If the ulcers prove resistant to treatment then bed rest with the feet elevated often promotes healing.

Apart from sensitisation to topical antibiotics there is a high degree of sensitisation in varicose eczema to other substances, such as lanolin, found in ointment bases, or to the ointment preservatives (Figure 5.8), and this should always be considered if the eczema shows no improvement or if it deteriorates, particularly with the spread of the eczema to other parts of the body. If sensitisation to any local medicaments is suspected, patch tests should be carried out.

### Surgery

In the very rare instance in which an ulcer shows no signs of healing, grafting may have to be considered. If the eczema is recurrent and/or long-standing and there are obvious varicose veins, a surgical opinion as to whether injection therapy or surgery would be helpful should be sought.

# 6. Seborrhoeic Eczema

THERE are two distinct types of eczema which may be considered under the heading of seborrhoeic eczema. One is the adult form which is most commonly seen in young and middle-aged adults, and the other the infantile variety which may begin as early as the age of six weeks, and is usually only present in infants under the age of eighteen months.

## Adult Seborrhoeic Eczema

Seborrhoeic eczema is one of the endogenous eczemas and the subdivision is based on purely clinical grounds. The term 'seborrhoeic' is somewhat misleading, because seborrhoea is not always present, and is certainly not required to make the diagnosis. However the sites commonly involved with this type of eczema are those areas of the skin where there are relatively more sebaceous glands per unit surface area i.e., face, scalp, and upper trunk. However, eczema occurring where two skin surfaces are in contact e.g. groins, axillae, peri-anal region, is considered to be a variant of seborrhoeic eczema and certainly at these sites there is not an increase of sebaceous glands per unit surface area.

As with other endogenous eczemas, the cause of seborrhoeic eczema is unknown, but there is often a positive family history. In the past, pyococcal infection of the skin was implicated as a possible cause, but the bacteria, if present, are now thought to colonise the skin as a secondary manifestation of the disorder. The term seborrhoeic dia-

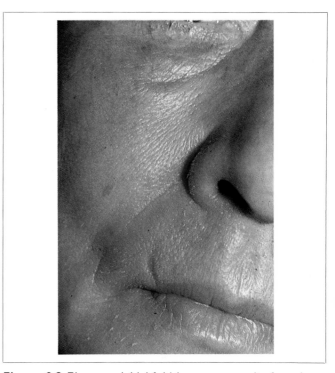

**Figure 6.2** *The naso-labial fold is a common site for seborrhoeic eczema.*

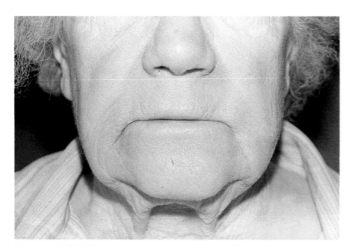

**Figure 6.1** *Seborrhoeic eczema at the sides of the nose and mouth.*

**Figure 6.3** (Right) *Confluent seborrhoeic eczema of the pinna.*

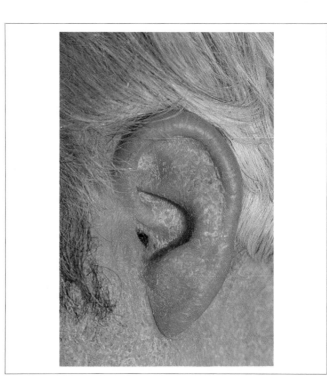

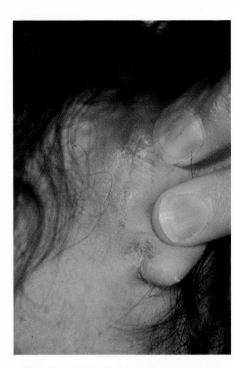

**Figure 6.4**
*Seborrhoeic
eczema behind
the ear, where
there may be
fissuring.*

thesis has also been used in the past and was meant to imply that subjects were prone to develop this type of eczema, but that it may occur at different sites at different times in their life. The term has now been dropped as it has very little meaning and does not contribute to our understanding of the disorder.

### Sites

There are three main distributional sub-types of seborrhoeic eczema. All or only one may be present.

1. The face, particularly the sides of the nose (Figure 6.1), naso-labial folds (Figure 6.2) and the chin (Figure 6.1); the scalp; the ears (Figure 6.3) and behind the ears (Figure 6.4) and around the eyelids (Figure 6.5). The eczema may be confluent or occur in small patches.

2. Presternal and interscapular areas of the trunk (Figures 6.6 and 6.7).

3. Intertrigo. This is a term used to denote seborrhoeic eczema occurring where two skin surfaces are in contact. The common factor appears to be perspiration which is unable to evaporate, keeping the area continuously moist. The common sites for this type of eczema are axillae (Figure 6.8), groins (Figure 6.9), submammary region in obese females (Figure 6.10), umbilicus and abdominal folds in obese persons (Figure 6.11), natal cleft and peri-anal skin (Figure 6.12), on the glans penis and under-surface of the foreskin (Figure 6.13).

### Morphology of Lesions

On the scalp the mildest seborrhoeic eczema is manifested by a diffuse scaling (*dandruff*). In more severe forms the scaling becomes thicker and at times may be difficult to distinguish from psoriasis of the scalp. In the most severe forms there is erythema, crusting and even exudation. Seborrhoeic eczema per se is not a cause of hair loss though the continual scratching may cause loss of hair, which is reversible.

When seborrhoeic eczema involves the pinnae or naso-labial folds it usually presents as redness and scaling (Figures 6.2 and 6.3), but in the later stages there may be fissuring above, below or behind the pinna (Figure 6.4). On the trunk seborrhoeic eczema occurs predominantly in the presternal and interscapular regions and the lesions are red and scaly (Figures 6.6 and 6.7). They may appear as small discs or annular lesions (Figure 6.7) and occasionally the eczema predominantly affects the hair follicles and presents as a follicular papular eruption.

### Intertrigo

When the eczema affects the intertriginous areas (Figures 6.8 to 6.13) (axillae, groins, submammary regions and umbilicus), the skin is red and sometimes macerated. In the natal cleft, particularly posteriorly, the skin may be fissured. In seborrhoeic eczema blistering and lichenification (thickening), present in other types of eczema of the skin, are not seen, and this may be a useful point in establishing the diagnosis.

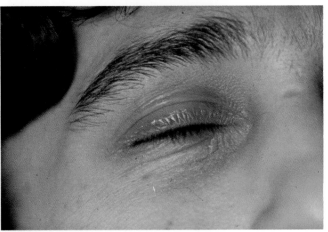

**Figure 6.5**
(Above)
*Seborrhoeic
eczema on the
eyelids and
surrounding skin.*

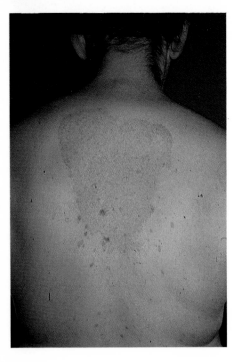

**Figure 6.6**
*Seborrhoeic
eczema in a
triangular pattern
between the
shoulder blades.*

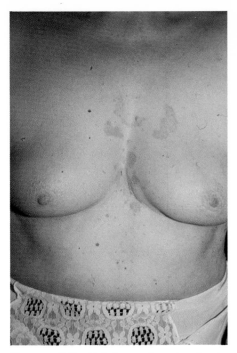

**Figure 6.7** *Patches of seborrhoeic eczema over the sternum.*

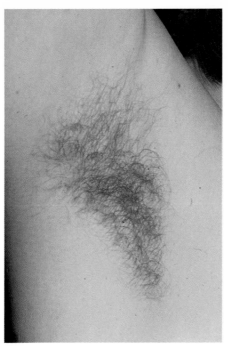

**Figure 6.8** *Patch of seborrhoeic eczema in the axilla.*

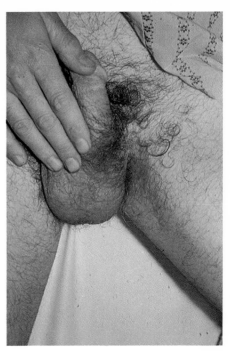

**Figure 6.9** *Eczema of the groin, thigh and scrotum where two skin surfaces are in contact.*

## Associated Conditions

Blepharitis (Figure 6.14) and otitis externa are often considered to be seborrhoeic eczema at specific sites and they may occur without eczema elsewhere. There is reported to be a higher incidence of acne and rosacea in patients who have or subsequently develop seborrhoeic eczema. However, there is no evidence as yet that one disorder causes the other.

## Natural History

Seborrhoeic eczema may be chronic and persistent or periodic. The exact cause is unknown but it is sometimes precipitated by overwork, lack of sleep and tension.

## Treatment

*Scalp.* In the mild forms of seborrhoeic eczema frequent shampooing may be all that is required. Patients should be reassured that frequent shampooing does not damage the hair or lead to baldness. The hair can be washed every two to three days. There are numerous shampoos which are advertised for the treatment of 'dandruff' but there is no specific shampoo which appears to reverse the process. The hair is often greasy in seborrhoeic eczema and frequently all that is required is a simple detergent shampoo. Strongly perfumed shampoos should not be used as they may act as irritants. Shampoos containing tar products may be helpful as the latter tend to suppress eczema.

If the condition is more severe with irritation, erythema and scaling of the scalp then a topical corticosteroid preparation will often reverse the eczematous process. Recently special vehicles for corticosteroid scalp applications have been formulated and they are more acceptable to patients than are ointments and creams.

**Figure 6.10** *Seborrhoeic eczema (intertriginous type) in submammary area. (Satellite lesions suggest secondary infection with monilia.)*

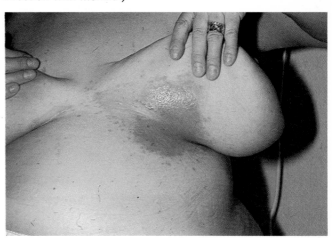

In the more severe chronic forms of scalp involvement with thick adherent scales a preparation containing keratolytics will be required. A suitable preparation is 2 per cent salicylic acid and 2 per cent sulphur in aqueous cream B.P. This should be applied two to three times a week at night and shampooed off the following morning. On the other nights a topical corticosteroid preparation mentioned above should be used.

*Face, pinnae and trunk.* At these sites topical corticosteroid preparations are the most effective treatment. Because the eczema tends to be moist, and often in exposed and visible areas, creams are often better and more acceptable than ointments. They should be applied at least twice a day. As

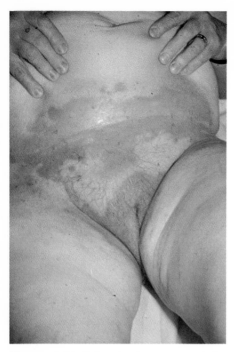

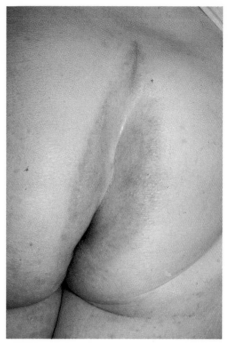

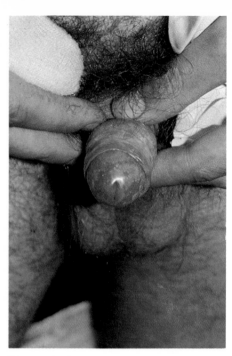

**Figure 6.11** *Seborrhoeic eczema of the abdominal fold, groins and skin of the vulva in an obese subject.*

**Figure 6.12** *Intertrigo in the natal cleft and on the peri-anal skin where skin surfaces are in contact.*

**Figure 6.13** *Intertrigo on glans penis.*

seborrhoeic eczema tends to be chronic in some patients the dangers of prolonged use of powerful topical corticosteroids must be appreciated, and those dangers are only now being realised. If these potent steroids are used over a period of two to three years there may be dermal and subcutaneous atrophy with the development of unsightly telangiectasia or striae (see Chapter 25). Thus in chronic cases it may be better to use the more potent corticosteroid preparations for only short periods, or to use a weaker steroid preparation such as 1 per cent hydrocortisone cream.

*Intertrigo.* There are two main aims in the management of intertrigo (a) to keep the area as dry as possible and (b) to counteract the eczema specifically. As the skin is moist and macerated there is often secondary infection with bacteria and/or fungi and to counteract this one should aim to keep the skin as dry as possible. Although not very acceptable cosmetically, the time honoured *pigmenta magenta* is highly effective in keeping the intertriginous area dry and counteracting secondary infection. The dye should be applied once a day, usually in the mornings, and at night a corticosteroid cream or lotion applied. Ointments are best avoided in intertriginous areas. It is particularly important to avoid the use of potent topical steroids in intertriginous areas for any length of time. The absorption of the steroid into the skin is greatly enhanced by the continuous moist conditions.

*Weight loss.* Obese subjects are more prone to develop intertrigo because opposing skin surfaces are more likely to be in contact. Thus in recurrent intertrigo weight loss should be advised.

*Antibiotics.* In practice topical corticosteroids per se will control seborrhoeic eczema, but secondary bacterial infec-

**Figure 6.14** *Blepharitis. Seborrhoeic eczema on the edges of the eyelids.*

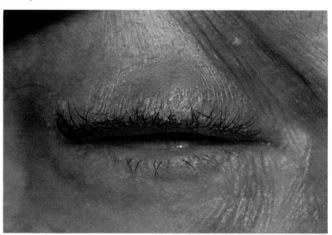

tion may occur, particularly in the intertriginous areas. The bacterial infection may be manifest by crusting or simply by resistance to treatment. Topical antibiotics such as neomycin and fusidic acid may be helpful combined with topical steroids. If there is no improvement with these antibiotics then swabs must be taken for culture and sensitivity of the organisms. It should also be remembered that monilia is a frequent secondary invader of intertrigo, and this is sometimes recognised as small satellite lesions (Figure 6.10). In these instances a preparation containing nystatin and a corticosteroid will be required.

*Systemic steroids.* As in other forms of endogenous eczema, systemic steroids should be reserved for the very severe or widespread forms of the disease which are not responding to topical measures. Fortunately such cases are extremely rare.

26

## Seborrhoeic Eczema of Infancy

Under this heading are a number of clinical entities seen in infancy. The term seborrhoeic eczema is used because the sites of involvement are the scalp and intertriginous areas. However, the disorder appears to be self-limiting and usually disappears by the age of two years. There does not appear to be a higher incidence of adult seborrhoeic eczema in later life.

### Cradle Cap

This may appear for the first time in infants a month old. In its mildest form it presents as yellow-brown greasy scaling on the scalp (Figure 6.15). The disorder is very common and tends to be self-limiting, clearing after six months. In its more severe forms the scales become thicker and heaped up presenting as thick, yellowish 'lumps' (Figure 6.16). In generalised seborrhoeic eczema of infancy the scalp may be red and scaly.

Corticosteroids are very rarely required for treating seborrhoeic eczema of the scalp, mild keratolytics are usually all that is needed. One per cent sulphur and one per cent salicylic acid in aqueous cream B.P. applied at night and shampooed out the next morning with a simple detergent shampoo is a simple and effective regime. In the more severe instances with thicker scales, the strength of keratolytics may be increased up to 5 per cent sulphur and 5 per cent salicylic acid.

### Nappy Rash

This is a very common disorder. It is arguable whether this should be considered as an exogenous eczema due to ammonia in the urine or as seborrhoeic eczema similar to intertrigo as seen in adults due to continual moisture of the skin. It would appear that some infants have a predisposition to eczema in the napkin area and this constitutional factor is probably the most important one. The eruption is usually confined to the napkin area (Figure 6.17), but like other eczemas there may be spread of the rash to other areas (see below). The diagnosis usually presents no difficulty. The rash in its mildest form is simply erythema. In the more severe forms there is exudation and even fissuring. A rarer manifestation of napkin eczema is a papular and vesicular eruption on the genitalia. Though diagnosis presents no difficulty, management does. As the disorder is due to moisture, or ammonia, or both, on the skin, the most appropriate treatment is to leave off the napkins. Most mothers, however, do not consider this practical advice and would find it impossible. A compromise may have to be reached in which the napkins are left off for short periods during the day, and the napkin changed at least once during the night. 'Nappy liners', which tend to keep the skin next to the liner drier than the napkin, should also be used. If these simple measures fail, then the eczema should be treated with 1 per cent hydrocortisone cream. As a rule potent topical steroids should not be used because of the increased absorption of steroid into the skin due to moisture and occlusion. Candida albicans is frequently found in napkin eczema, probably as a secondary disorder, although

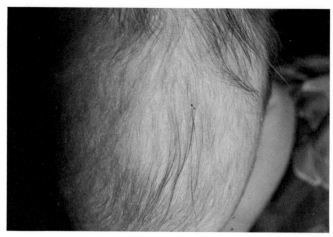

**Figure 6.15** *Cradle cap. Yellowish-brown scaling in seborrhoeic eczema of the scalp in infancy.*

**Figure 6.16** *Thick 'lumpy' yellowish scaly lesion in seborrhoeic eczema of the scalp.*

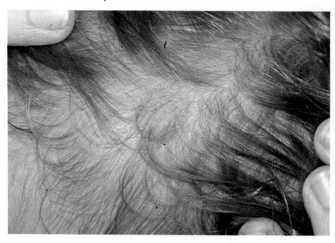

**Figure 6.17** *Nappy rash. The rash is confined to the napkin area.*

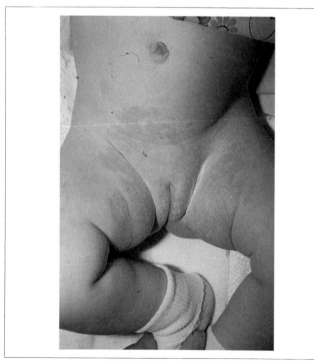

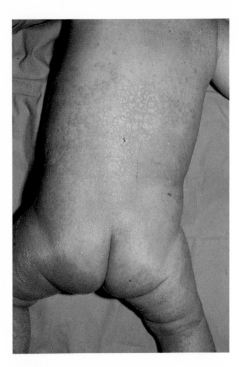

**Figure 6.18**
*Confluent erythema spreading from the napkin area to the trunk in generalised seborrhoeic eczema of infancy.*

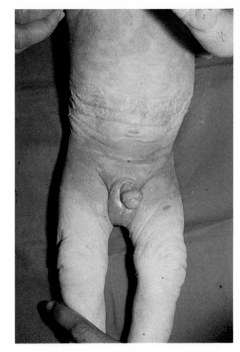

**Figure 6.20**
*Severe seborrhoeic eczema of infancy. The lesions outside the napkin area show scaling similar to that of psoriasis.*

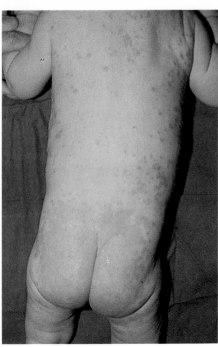

**Figure 6.19**
*Small red scaly patches on the trunk in another form of generalised seborrhoeic eczema of infancy.*

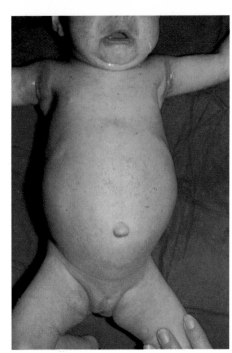

**Figure 6.21**
*Spread of seborrhoeic eczema of infancy to the axillae.*

there are those who consider that it plays a role in the production of the eruption. Occasionally, better results of treatment can be obtained by combining nystatin with the hydrocortisone.

### Generalised Seborrhoeic Eczema of Infancy

This eruption usually begins as a napkin eczema. However, the eczema then appears outside the napkin area. The eruption outside the napkin area may take one of two forms or appear as a combination of both. First, there is extension of eczema from the napkin area on to the trunk and down the thighs. This may spread as a confluent erythema (Figure 6.18) or as small red patches (Figure 6.19).

Not infrequently these lesions develop a white scaly surface as seen in psoriasis (Figure 6.20), and the term napkin psoriasis has been used to describe this eruption. However, this term is probably best avoided because there is no evidence that these infants have a higher incidence of psoriasis in later life, and the prognosis of generalised seborrhoeic eczema of infancy is excellent, the rash clearing permanently once the infants are out of napkins. The second type of spread seen in generalised seborrhoeic eczema of infancy is confluent erythema in other intertriginous areas, e.g. axillae (Figure 6.21) and neck (Figure 6.22). The face (Figure 6.23) is frequently involved in this type of eczema and may in fact be the first site to be affected.

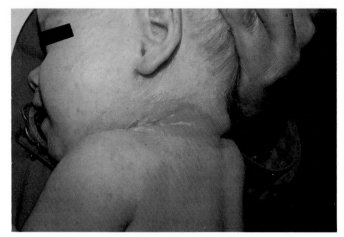

**Figure 6.22** *Severe exudative eczema of the intertriginous skin of the neck in seborrhoeic eczema of infancy.*

The cause of the spread of the eczema in generalised seborrhoeic eczema is not known. As in napkin eczema, candida albicans infection has been implicated, but there is no conclusive evidence that this organism is the sole cause.

Treatment of generalised seborrhoeic eczema of infancy is similar to that of napkin eczema. Weak topical steroid creams, such as 1 per cent hydrocortisone, possibly combined with nystatin, should be applied three times a day. If there is no satisfactory response, then the strength of steroid cream may be cautiously increased, but this should probably be left to a specialist.

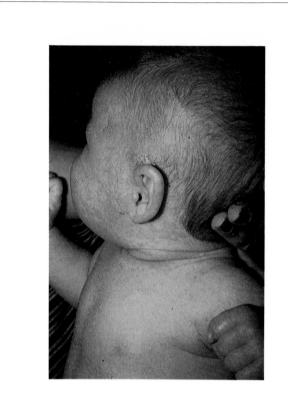

**Figure 6.23** *The face is commonly affected in seborrhoeic eczema of infancy.*

# 7. Nummular Eczema and Pompholyx Eczema

### Nummular Eczema

THIS pattern of endogenous eczema is sometimes referred to as discoid eczema. There are no known definite aetiological factors, and like many other skin disorders the name is based on purely descriptive grounds.

### Morphology of Lesions

The lesions of nummular eczema occur mainly on the extensor surfaces of the limbs and the eruption tends to be (Figures 7.1 and 7.2), vesicles and exudation (Figure 7.3). The lesions may coalesce to form large confluent areas of eczema (Figure 7.3) or small satellite lesions may develop around the original lesion (Figure 7.4).

### Distribution

The lesions of nummular eczema occur mainly on the extensor surfaces of the limbs and the eruption tends to be distributed symmetrically (Figures 7.3 and 7.5). Certain localised areas may be involved, such as the nipples, or the dorsa of the hands (Figure 7.5). The individual number of patches when the eczema involves these sites varies from a few to many. Like any other pattern of eczema, nummular eczema may occasionally become extensive and generalised, possibly due to auto sensitisation.

### Age Incidence and Natural History

Nummular eczema seldom affects people under 20. It seems commonest in young and middle-aged adults, but it does occur in elderly persons, particularly those with dry skins. The eczema usually lasts for a period of several months, but eventually tends to clear. The relapse rate does not appear to be as high as in other types of endogenous eczema e.g. atopic or seborrhoeic.

### Management and Treatment

In the acute stages of nummular eczema, if there is exudation, lotions and compresses will have to be applied, and the affected areas covered with clean linen dressings. Potassium permanganate soaks 1:10,000 or physiological saline should be used in the first instance. As the lesions become drier a steroid cream should be used. A moderately potent topical steroid should be used initially. The cream should be

**Figure 7.1** *Localised patch of nummular eczema. The eczema is subacute with crusting.*

**Figure 7.2** *Areas of nummular eczema on the dorsum of the hand.*

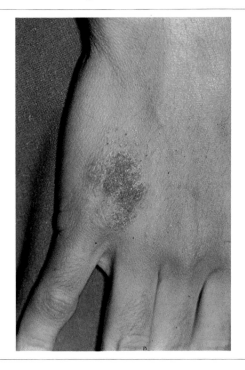

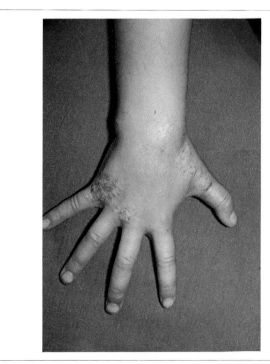

applied at least twice a day, and the affected part subsequently covered by tube-gauze dressings, or cotton gloves for the hands. In the more chronic phase a steroid ointment should be used. The strength of topical steroid will depend on the initial response. If the disorder is easily suppressed the patient may be given a supply of the steroid and instructed to use it if there is a relapse. If the condition proves difficult to suppress then a short course of a very potent topical steroid would be justified. If it is necessary to give maintenance treatment for a prolonged period of time, e.g. months, then it is advisable to dilute the more powerful topical steroids.

*Antibiotics.* Like any other eczema there is always a possibility of secondary infection with pathogenic organisms.

The lesions may become frankly purulent or impetiginised i.e. have yellow crusts. In these circumstances a local antibiotic will be required. Neomycin or fusidic acid ointment is usually adequate to control the infection but if there is no improvement after two or three days a swab should be taken and the appropriate topical antibiotic given as determined by the swab report. Systemic antibiotics will be required if there is evidence of spread of the infection.

*Systemic steroids.* Fortunately these are only very rarely required to control this type of eczema, and should never be used as a first measure.

*Baths.* Nummular eczema has sometimes been attributed to too frequent bathing particularly with antiseptics and toilet

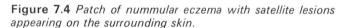

**Figure 7.3** *Acute symmetrical nummular eczema on the extensor surfaces of the forearms.*

**Figure 7.4** *Patch of nummular eczema with satellite lesions appearing on the surrounding skin.*

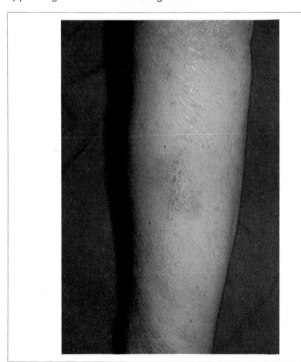

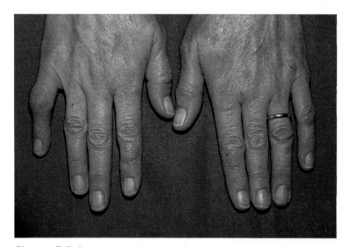

**Figure 7.5** *Symmetrical nummular eczema on the dorsa of the hands.*

**Figure 7.6** *Symmetrical eruption of pompholyx eczema on the soles of the feet.*

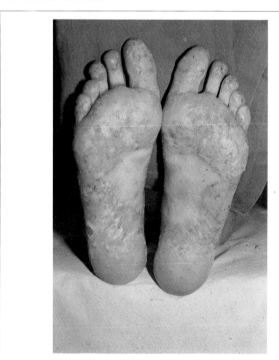

preparations added to the bath water. These added substances should therefore be avoided and a mild emollient, such as Ung. Emulsificans B.P. should be applied after bathing.

## Pompholyx Eczema

This type of eczema occurs on the hands and feet, and the name is taken from the Greek word *pompholyx* which means 'bubble' as the disorder is characterised by numerous blisters. If the eczema is confined to the hands it is sometimes referred to as cheiropompholyx, and if confined to the feet as podopompholyx. Another term sometimes applied to this form of eczema is 'dyshidrotic' as the eczema appears to be aggravated by excessive sweating of the palms and soles.

### Distribution

Pompholyx eczema affects the hands and feet (Figure 7.6) either together or separately. The hands are more commonly involved. The eczema tends to affect those areas involved by emotional sweating, i.e. on the hands—the palms, sides of fingers, and the dorsal aspects of the fingers over the distal two phalanges, and on the feet—the soles and sides of the toes. As with the fingers the dorsal surface of the toes over the distal phalanges may be involved. The eruption tends to be symmetrical (Figures 7.6 and 7.7), whether it is the hands or feet which are affected. Pompholyx eczema, like other forms of eczema, may spread from the palms and soles to affect other areas of the body. Initially the eczema spreads to affect the back of the hands (Figure 7.8) and then up the arms (Figure 7.9), and may even give rise to a generalised eruption.

### Type of Lesion

The characteristic lesion is the blister, and this varies in size from 1 mm to 1 cm or even larger (Figures 7.7, 7.10 and 7.11). The small blisters are the commoner type of lesion. There may be only a few blisters or they may be very numerous and involve the entire palm and sides of fingers. Because the keratin layer is so thick on the palm and sole the blisters (although epidermal) do not rupture immediately and they appear as small firm white lesions (Figure 7.10). The blisters may eventually rupture and the skin break down and present an exuding or crusted surface (Figures 7.6 and 7.9) or the blisters may resolve slowly, the fluid being reabsorbed into the circulation with no break in the skin surface. The blisters frequently occur in groups on the palms, and the whole palm is not necessarily involved (Figure 7.7). Occasionally only the sides of the fingers and not the palms are affected. If only the dorsal aspect of the fingers are involved, the condition may be confused with other types of eczema. In the more chronic forms of the disorder, no blisters may be seen but the eczema presents as scaling and fissuring on the palms (Figures 7.12 and 7.13) and soles which may be difficult to heal.

### Natural History and Precipitating Factors

The disorder is rare in early childhood, but can occur at any age. The eczema tends to occur in 'attacks' and run a self-limiting two to four-week course. Occasionally the disorder becomes chronic and new blisters appear as the old ones clear. Alternatively, the patient may have one or many episodes during a year, and then may be free for a number of years. Frequently the attacks are precipitated by warm

**Figure 7.7** *Symmetrical pompholyx eczema on the palms, presenting as small blisters.*

**Figure 7.8** *Chronic pompholyx eczema which has spread to involve the backs of the hands and wrists.*

**Figure 7.9** *Subacute pompholyx eczema on the palms spreading to the forearms. The blisters have ruptured and there is crust formation.*

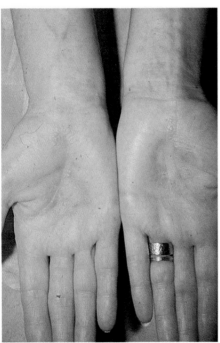

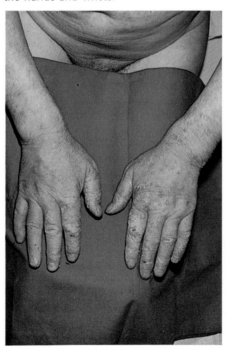

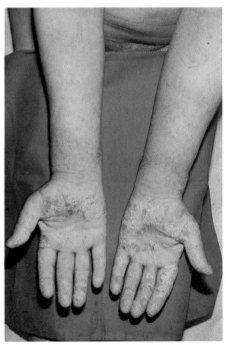

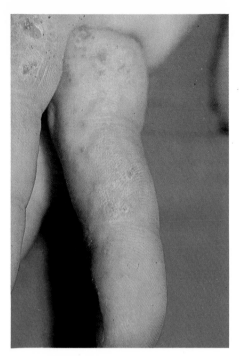

**Figure 7.10**
*Typical small blisters of pompholyx eczema on the sides of the fingers. Some of the blisters have ruptured.*

weather and helped by cooler weather. The other known precipitating factor is emotional stress which is thought to induce the attacks by increased perspiration on the palms and soles.

## Management and Treatment

In the early stages when the blisters first appear there is usually intense irritation, and antipruritics such as promethazine or trimeprazine are helpful. Both these drugs tend to cause drowsiness about which patients must be warned, but because of this side-effect they are very good for use at night as they tend to promote sleep.

*Soaks.* If the blisters are rupturing and there is exudation, warm potassium permanganate soaks 1:8,000 should be given for 10 to 15 minutes four times a day. Potassium permanganate is probably the most effective solution in which to soak the affected parts but it has the slight disadvantage of staining the skin and nails brown (Figure 7.14).

*Corticosteroids.* In the acute stages 1 per cent hydrocortisone cream is probably all that is required. This should be applied

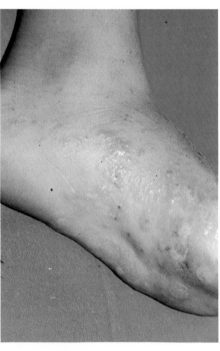

**Figure 7.11**
*Blisters of varying size on the sole in pompholyx eczema.*

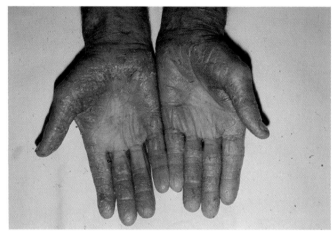

**Figure 7.13** *Symmetrical thick hyperkeratotic scaling and fissures in the chronic type of pompholyx eczema.*

**Figure 7.14** *Brownish-purple discoloration of the nails and skin due to potassium permanganate soaks.*

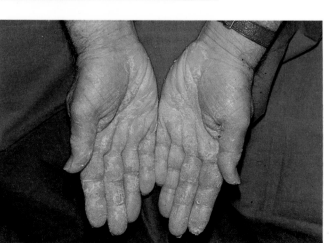

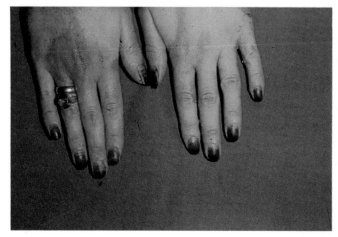

**Figure 7.12** (Left) *Chronic stage of pompholyx eczema, only erythema and hyperkeratotic scaling are seen.*

after the potassium permanganate soaks. In the subacute and chronic stages the more powerful topical corticosteroid preparations should be used. Unfortunately, topical corticosteroids do not appear to be helpful in preventing further attacks, and play no part in prophylaxis.

Systemic corticosteroids may shorten an attack of pompholyx eczema but since most attacks are self-limiting their use is probably not justified. In the chronic forms of the disease there is usually relapse when the steroids are withdrawn, so they are probably best avoided in the first place.

*Antibiotics.* Pompholyx eczema not infrequently becomes infected and may present as pustules as opposed to blisters. In these instances there may be lymphangitis or cellulitis if the affecting organism is a streptococcus, and systemic antibiotics should be given. If the secondary infection is more superficial and presents as crusts, then topical antibiotics, either fusidic acid or neomycin, combined with the topical corticosteroid should be used until the infection has cleared.

*Dressings.* In the acute stages the affected hands and feet should be covered with clean linen dressings and the limb rested. In the subacute and chronic stages cotton gloves or socks should be used.

*General advice.* As has already been stated there is no certain way of preventing further attacks. If the attacks are precipitated by emotional problems these should be dealt with and the patient may benefit from the appropriate psychotropic drugs. If the attacks are precipitated by heat this should be avoided if possible, and when the feet are affected cotton socks are preferable to nylon or woollen ones.

# 8. Psoriasis

PSORIASIS is a common skin disorder, and it has been estimated that it affects approximately two per cent of Caucasians at some stage during their lives.

## Aetiology

The exact cause of psoriasis is unknown. One-third of patients with this complaint give a history of psoriasis in a blood relative. It is thought that there is a specific inherited defect in the skin which allows psoriasis to develop under certain circumstances. There are a number of known factors which precipitate or aggravate psoriasis.

(a) Streptococcal infections. Psoriasis sometimes first appears two to three weeks after a streptococcal infection. The mechanism is unknown.

(b) Mental stress. Psoriasis is not *caused* by mental stress but in persons with the probable inherited defect in the skin, worry may precipitate psoriasis for the first time, or aggravate it in one who already has the disease.

(c) Trauma. Trauma to the skin can induce lesions in some patients with psoriasis.

(d) Drugs. Chloroquine can sometimes precipitate or aggravate psoriasis.

## Age Incidence

Psoriasis is extremely rare in those under the age of five years. It is uncommon between the ages of five and ten but does occur. The commonest age at which it first appears is between fifteen and thirty years. The incidence of 'first attack' then falls progressively with advancing years, but psoriasis may appear for the first time in the eighth and ninth decades.

## Natural History

Psoriasis tends to be a chronic disorder. The extent and chronicity of lesions vary greatly from patient to patient. In a recent survey of over 2,000 patients, 38.5 per cent reported a remission in their disease at some stage, including spontaneous remissions and those induced by treatment. The length of time remissions last is variable. Those induced by therapy vary according to the drug used.

**Figure 8.1** *Typical lesion of psoriasis. Well-demarcated plaque showing silvery-white scales.*

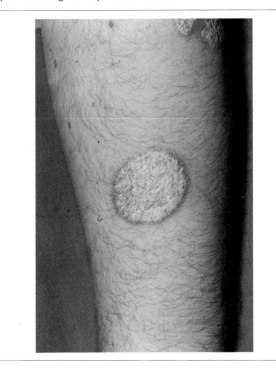

**Figure 8.2** *Two psoriatic lesions. The lower lesion is a red plaque with minimal scaling; the upper lesion initially had a similar appearance but after excoriation the typical white scales of psoriasis were produced.*

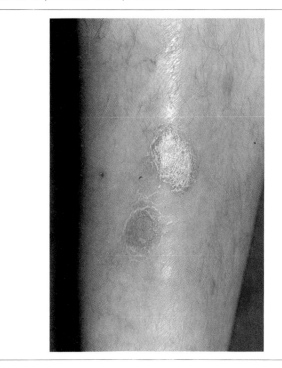

Remissions induced by tar or dithranol preparations tend to be longer than those induced by topical corticosteroids. Occasionally remissions are permanent, or at least may last for several years. Why psoriasis remits in some patients but not in others even with the same treatment is as yet unknown. Psoriasis is a disorder which has varying degrees of activity. If the disease is very active then the eruption is extensive and the relapse rate after treatment is rapid, irrespective of treatment. If the activity is moderate then a reasonable period of remission can be expected after treatment. If the degree of activity is low, spontaneous remis-

sions occur and may be long-lasting. It is not possible at present to estimate the degree of activity of psoriasis.

## Clinical Presentation

Psoriasis is usually easy to diagnose on clinical grounds but occasionally diagnosis can be extremely difficult because of varied presentations.

## Distribution and Morphology

The classical lesion of psoriasis is a raised, red, scaly, circular or oval plaque whose edges are sharply marginated

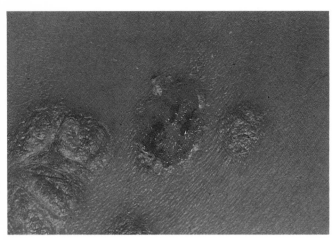

**Figure 8.3** *Capillary bleeding points in a psoriatic lesion after removal of the scales.*

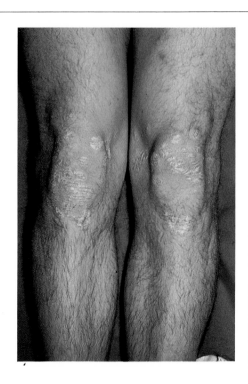

**Figure 8.4** (Right) *Typical symmetrical lesions of psoriasis on the knees.*

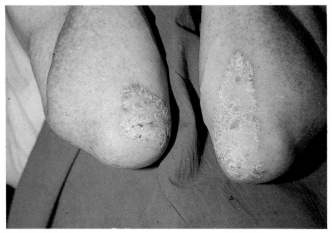

**Figure 8.5** *Psoriasis on the elbows, one of the commonest sites.*

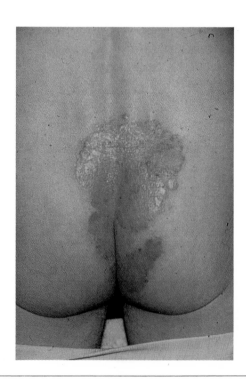

**Figure 8.6** (Right) *Plaque of psoriasis over the sacrum.*

(Figure 8.1). Occasionally it has a geographic pattern. The *scaling* tends to be silvery or white (Figure 8.1). Sometimes this type of scaling is not present and the lesion presents as a red plaque. If the diagnosis of psoriasis is suspected the lesion should be gently excoriated with a wooden spatula and if it is psoriasis the white silvery scale will appear (Figure 8.2). Further confirmation can be obtained if all the scale is removed, when a red, smooth, slightly moist area will be revealed with capillary bleeding points (Figure 8.3). The commonest sites to be involved in psoriasis are the knees (Figure 8.4) and elbows (Figure 8.5). Next commonest are the sacral area (Figure 8.6) and the scalp behind the ears. It is important to examine all sites if a diagnosis of psoriasis is suspected.

*Trunk and limbs.* Psoriasis on the trunk and limbs may present in a number of ways. It may appear as discoid or oval patches (Figures 8.4 and 8.5), which can vary in size from one to ten cm with completely normal looking skin in between. In the more severe forms the plaques become more numerous (Figure 8.7) and larger (Figure 8.8), and eventually become confluent (Figure 8.9). Very occasionally the whole of the skin surface may become involved, so-called *erythrodermic psoriasis.* In this form of the disease the skin may not have the typical white silvery scales of psoriasis, but presents a generalised erythema with superficial scaling (Figure 8.10) which may be indistinguishable from erythroderma due to eczema. Another presentation is numerous small red papules which still have the classical scale if excoriated. These appear suddenly on trunk and limbs. This presentation is sometimes referred to as *guttate psoriasis* (Figures 8.11 and 8.12). This is the usual pattern that appears after a streptococcal infection. Guttate

psoriasis tends to have a good prognosis and often clears spontaneously within three months.

*Scalp.* Involvement of the scalp is fairly common. It may occur with the disease affecting the skin at other sites but occasionally it affects *only* the scalp and the diagnosis may then be difficult on clinical grounds alone. As with the skin elsewhere psoriasis may involve the whole of the scalp or only small areas. The scales on the scalp lesions tend to be heaped up so that they feel 'lumpy' and irregular (sometimes referred to as 'rocks') and often the diagnosis is made by palpation as well as inspection (Figure 8.13). Psoriasis of the scalp usually stops at the hair line and does not spread on to the neck or face in the majority of patients (Figures 8.14 and 8.15).

*Intertriginous areas.* If psoriasis affects the skin in the groins, axillae (Figure 8.16), peri-anal region (Figure 8.17), between the toes, or under the breasts or the umbilicus (Figure 8.18), the appearances differ from the classical raised red plaque with silvery white scales. Where the skin surfaces are in opposition and the areas are moist, there is no dry scale and the lesions present as smooth confluent red plaques, which may or may not be raised. Occasionally, particularly between the toes, the scale which is present has a macerated appearance, which used to be called 'white' psoriasis.

*Palms and soles.* There are two different types of psoriasis affecting the palms and soles. Neither has the classical appearances of psoriasis and, if localised only to these sites, may give rise to difficulty in diagnosis. First it may present as localised areas of erythema, scaling and fissuring, tending to be symmetrical (Figures 8.19 and 8.20). Like

**Figure 8.7** *Numerous plaques of psoriasis on the back in active psoriasis.*

**Figure 8.8** *Large plaques of psoriasis on the buttocks and back.*

**Figure 8.9** *Confluent thick plaque of psoriasis on the back at a chronic stage of the disorder.*

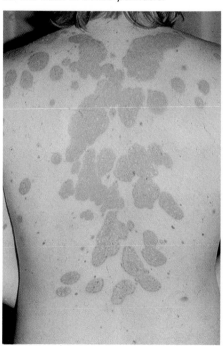
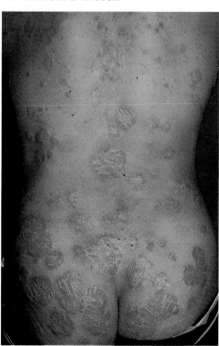
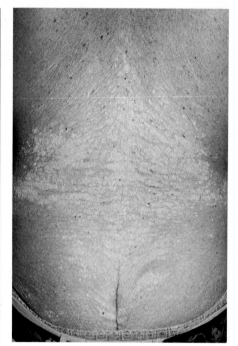

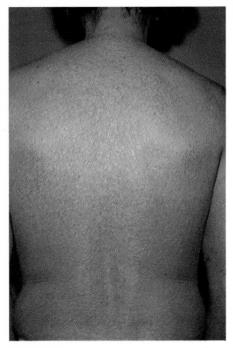

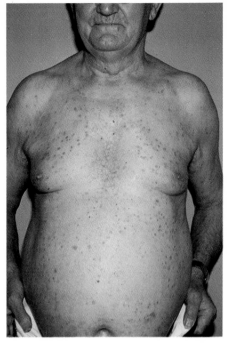

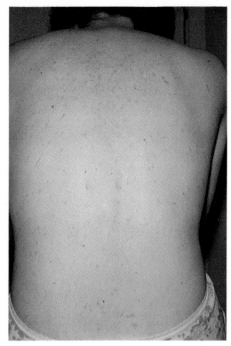

**Figure 8.10** *Erythrodermic psoriasis.*

**Figure 8.11** *Numerous small red papules of psoriasis. The pattern is often referred to as guttate psoriasis.*

**Figure 8.12** *Guttate psoriasis. The typical white scaling may be absent but can be produced by excoriation.*

**Figure 8.13** *Thick scales of psoriasis on the scalp.*

**Figure 8.14** *Typical silvery-white scales of psoriasis on the scalp. The disorder tends to stop at the hair-line.*

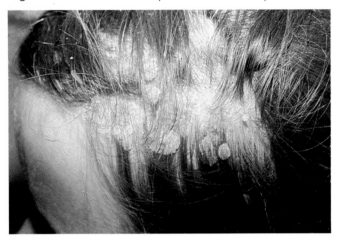

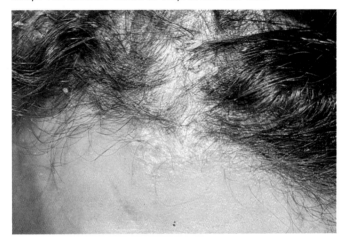

psoriasis elsewhere there is often a sharp line of demarcation between the affected and unaffected skin (Figure 8.21). The appearances are sometimes difficult to distinguish from chronic eczema of the palms and soles. The second manifestation of psoriasis affecting the palms and soles is termed *pustular psoriasis*. However, it is not certain whether this disorder is truly psoriasis or whether it represents a separate disease entity. The other terms sometimes used for this condition are persistent palmar and plantar pustulosis or recalcitrant eruption of the palms and soles. Pustular psoriasis presents as discrete red scaly areas on the palms and soles and small sterile pustules are present (Figures 8.22 and 8.23). The disorder may be symmetrical or occasionally only affects one palm or sole. As some of the terms applied to this condition imply, the disorder tends

to be very persistent and may last for years. Typical psoriatic lesions elsewhere on the skin are present in less than 20 per cent of patients with pustular psoriasis.

*Nails.* The nails are frequently involved in psoriasis and this may be helpful in establishing the diagnosis, if the nature of the skin eruption is in doubt. The nails are involved in psoriasis in three ways:

(a) The nails show small pits (Figure 8.24) with wide variation in the number of pits present.

(b) The terminal part of the nail plate separates from the nail bed (onycholysis) so that the distal part of the nail appears white (Figure 8.25). Occasionally the area under the nail plate proves a suitable place to harbour chromo-

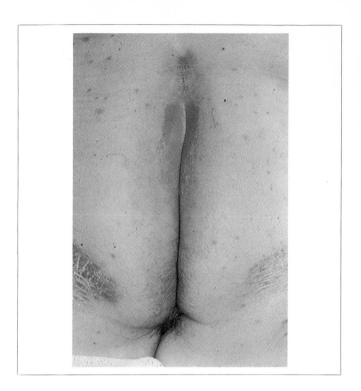

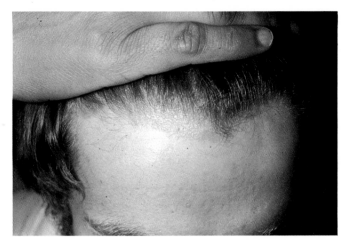

**Figure 8.15** *Psoriasis of the scalp. The disease usually stops at, or just beyond, the hair-line.*

**Figure 8.16** *Psoriasis localised to the axilla—intertriginous psoriasis.*

**Figure 8.18** *Intertriginous psoriasis around and in the umbilicus.*

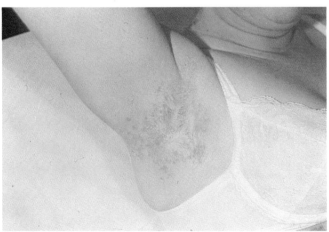

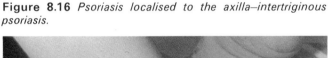

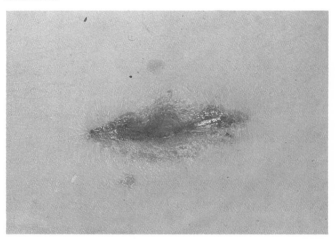

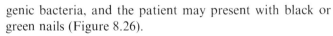

genic bacteria, and the patient may present with black or green nails (Figure 8.26).

(c) The nail plate becomes thickened and there is thick scale (hyperkeratosis) under the nail plate (Figure 8.27).

Occasionally psoriasis affects only the nails and there are no skin lesions. In these circumstances the diagnosis can be extremely difficult to establish, and particularly to distinguish from a fungus infection if the involvement causes thickening of the nail plate with subungual hyperkeratosis. In psoriasis occasionally, but not always, all the nails are involved, but in a fungus infection only a few (at least at the onset) are involved. In order to try to establish the diagnosis, specimens of the nail should be taken for culture and microscopy to determine whether fungus is present.

*Arthritis.* Approximately five per cent of patients with psoriasis develop an arthritis, which is distinguished from rheumatoid arthritis by the absence of the 'rheumatoid factor' in the serum. Psoriatic arthritis is therefore sometimes referred to as 'sero-negative' arthritis. The joints of the hand are frequently affected but unlike rheumatoid arthritis, the terminal interphalangeal joint may be involved (Figures 8.28 and 8.29), as well as the other joints of the fingers and hand (Figure 8.30). The knee and ankle joints are also commonly affected. Occasionally 'psoriatic arthropathy' occurs without the skin lesions of psoriasis. Under these circumstances the diagnosis will have to be made by the clinical features, the absence of the rheumatoid factor in the serum, the exclusion of other causes of arthropathy

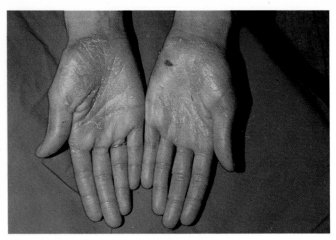

**Figure 8.19** *Psoriasis on the palms presenting as symmetrical, red, scaly lesions with fissuring. If there are no psoriatic lesions elsewhere, the diagnosis may be difficult to make.*

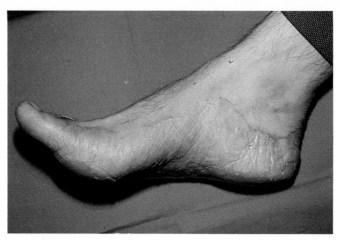

**Figure 8.21** *Sharp line of demarcation between the affected and unaffected skin on the sole of the foot. This point may help in making the diagnosis.*

**Figure 8.20** *Symmetrical erythema, scaling and fissuring in psoriasis on the soles.*

**Figure 8.22** *Pustular psoriasis. Scaling and pustules in a localised area on the sole.*

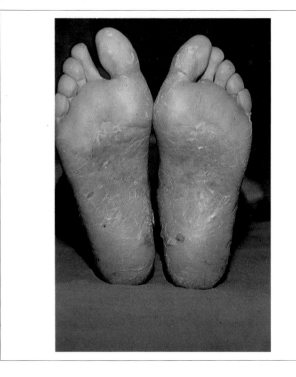

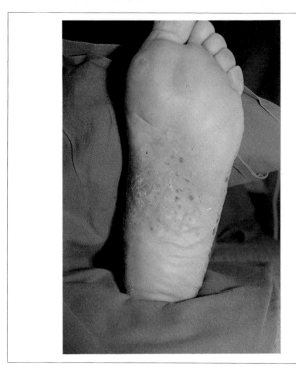

such as gout and systemic lupus erythematosus, and possibly a family history of psoriasis.

The treatment of psoriatic arthritis is similar to that of rheumatoid arthritis. Salicylates, phenylbutazone and indomethacin are all useful drugs. Systemic steroids should be avoided if possible as they make control of the skin lesions more difficult, for when the dose of steroid is reduced there is frequently a flare-up of the lesions.

### Treatment and Management

Once the diagnosis of psoriasis has been made it is most important that certain features of the disorder are explained to the patient before embarking on any form of treatment. First, the patient must be reassured that the disorder is not contagious and that it is not a sign of any internal disease. It should be explained that psoriasis does not, in itself, have any serious systemic effects.

Patients will often ask about the cause of psoriasis, and they must be given an explanation of their disease. With our present knowledge patients can be told that they have a (probably hereditary) defect in the skin which under certain circumstances will cause the skin to develop into a psoriatic lesion. However, they should also be reassured that just as psoriasis may appear for the first time after thirty or forty years of life so it may well disappear for no apparent reason. They should also be told that when psoriasis clears it does not leave any marks or scars and the skin returns to a normal appearance. It is, however, only fair to tell the

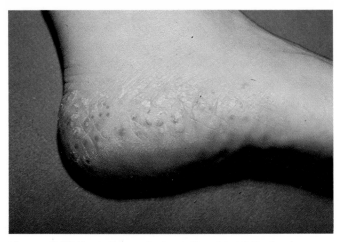

**Figure 8.23** *Pustular psoriasis on the side of the heel.*

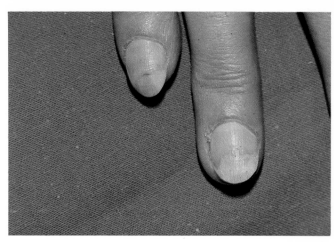

**Figure 8.25** *Onycholysis, separation of the distal part of the nail plate from the nail bed.*

**Figure 8.24** *Typical pits in psoriasis affecting the nail plate.*

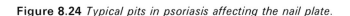

**Figure 8.26** *Onycholysis with chromogenic bacteria producing a green colour under the nail plate.*

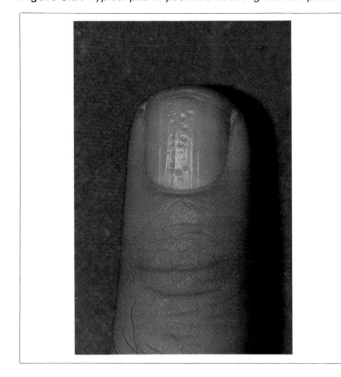

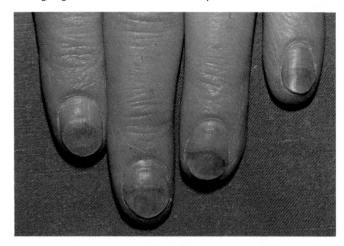

patients that at the present time there is no known *permanent* cure for the disorder but that something can always be done to improve the condition, even if the effects are not long-lasting. Patients should also be told that psoriasis can always be cleared by intensive therapy but that when the lesions do clear, either spontaneously or as a result of treatment, then the length of remission cannot be foretold, though it could be permanent.

Finally, each patient must be regarded individually. Some patients who have minimal psoriasis and who have had the nature of the condition explained, will be perfectly satisfied to receive no treatment, but others with the same involvement will demand vigorous treatment to try to clear the condition. Whatever course is finally adopted the doctor

must be sure the treatment being given is not worse than the disease he is trying to clear, which often happens with psoriatic patients.

### Topical Measures

Psoriasis being a 'benign' condition, the treatments most commonly employed are topical measures rather than systemic therapy, but even topical treatments are not without side-effects and these must be fully appreciated.

### Topical Corticosteroids

Unfortunately the treatment of psoriasis, unlike eczema, has not been transformed with the advent of the new powerful topical corticosteroids, although it has been helped. The mechanism of action of topical steroids in psoriasis is not known at the present time.

*Indications for topical corticosteroids.* If psoriasis is particularly acute with new lesions appearing, or in the erythrodermic stage, corticosteroids are usually the most appropriate topical measure. They are also indicated and effective for psoriasis in the groins, axillae, and on the face. They are probably effective in intertriginous areas because of greater

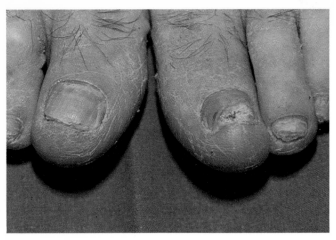

**Figure 8.27** *Thickening of the nail plate and subungual hyperkeratosis in psoriasis.*

**Figure 8.28** *Psoriatic arthritis. The proximal interphalangeal joint of the index finger and the terminal interphalangeal joint of the little finger are affected.*

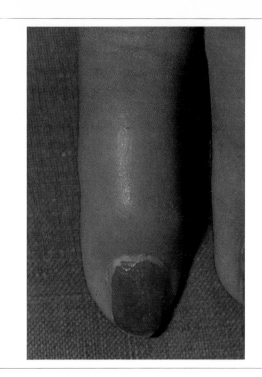

**Figure 8.29** *Arthropathy of the terminal interphalangeal joint in psoriasis (this does not occur in rheumatoid arthritis).*

**Figure 8.30** *Severe deformity of the hands due to psoriatic arthropathy.*

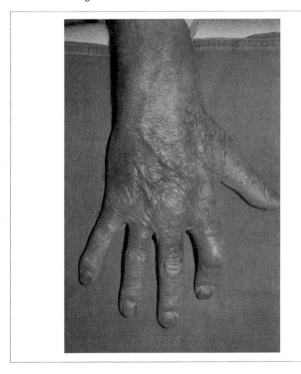

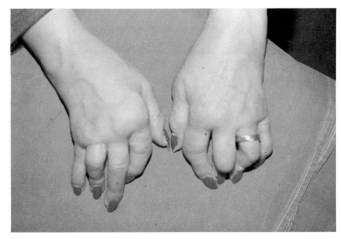

absorption of the steroid in these moist areas, and also in psoriasis on the face as the skin is thinner and, once again, more of the active substance may be absorbed. As a rule creams rather than ointments should be used for intertriginous areas.

Topical steroids are often helpful for the chronic plaque of psoriasis and are probably the treatment of first choice because of their simplicity and cosmetic acceptability. As a rule, the more potent the topical steroid the more effective it is in clearing psoriasis. Thus the most potent topical steroid available at present (clobetasol propionate) is more effective than the weaker topical steroids. However, it must be stressed that the greater the strength of the steroid, the greater the incidence of side-effects. Clobetasol propionate

should not be used for periods longer than two weeks at a time, and with an interval of two months between courses of treatment. Also clobetasol propionate should not be used in the intertriginous areas or on the face.

Intermediate strength topical steroids are often used and are helpful as a long term measure in controlling the extent of psoriasis without actually clearing the lesions. However, if these preparations are used for any length of time the patient must be seen at regular intervals to be assessed for possible side effects. Repeat prescriptions issued over months or years without seeing the patient's skin are not acceptable. In dealing with topical steroids it is again stressed that side effects tend to be proportional to the product of the duration of use and strength of steroid.

*Polythene occlusive dressings.* Topical steroids used under polythene occlusive dressings are now not used as often as previously. There is no doubt that the effect of the steroid is enhanced when used in this manner but the more potent topical steroids are often effective without polythene dressings. Treatment with polythene dressings should now probably be reserved for short periods as a 'special' treatment for clearing persistent plaque lesions for particular occasions, e.g. prior to a holiday. Only small areas should be treated with these dressings at one time, and the dressings should be used only for a 12 hour period each day. Treatment should not be continued for longer than two weeks.

*Disadvantages and side effects of topical corticosteroids.* The main disadvantage of topical corticosteroids is the high relapse rate when the treatment is stopped, but they are far more cosmetically acceptable to the patients than are tar or dithranol compounds. Side effects of topical steroids are dealt with in detail in Chapter 25, but they are mentioned here because it is important to be aware of them.

*Striae.* If the steroids are used for any length of time, in the intertriginous areas or under occlusive dressings where the absorption of the steroid is increased, then striae, similar to those seen in Cushing's disease, may develop. These tend to be permanent and for this reason it is inadvisable to use such preparations indefinitely, particularly under the conditions mentioned above.

*Subcutaneous and collagen atrophy.* Wasting of the subcutaneous tissues and atrophy of the connective tissues of the dermis may occur after the prolonged use of the more potent topical steroids. It is far more likely to occur if the steroids are used under polythene occlusive dressings. Apart from the skin appearing thinner, atrophy of the collagen of the skin presents as spontaneous bruising.

*Secondary infection.* Psoriasis does not usually become secondarily infected, but when the skin is covered with polythene the increase in temperature and humidity predisposes to infection of the *normal* skin which is also covered with these dressings.

### Tar Preparations

There are many tar preparations available for the treatment of psoriasis but the most effective is 5 per cent crude coal tar in Lassar's paste. The more purified tar preparations in a pleasant creamy base, although more cosmetically acceptable to the patient, are not so effective.

Tar preparations are more effective when used in conjunction with ultra-violet light, and at present this regime is usually practical only for in-patient therapy.

The 5 per cent crude coal tar should be applied to the lesions daily (except those on the face and scalp) and the affected part of the body is then covered with tube-gauze dressings. After 24 hours the tar paste should be removed in a bath to which has been added 30 ml coal tar solution B.P. Following the bath, a suberythema dose of ultra-violet light should be given. The whole procedure is then

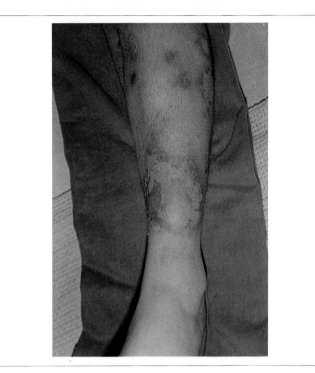

**Figure 8.31** *Staining of 'normal' skin around psoriatic lesions which have been treated with dithranol. There is no staining of the skin of the lesion itself.*

**Figure 8.32** *Severe irritant reaction in the 'normal' skin with blister formation due to dithranol.*

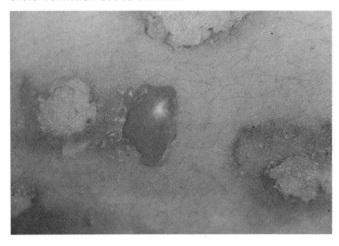

repeated for three to four weeks, by which time clearing of the lesions should have been obtained.

*Disadvantages of tar therapy.* The main disadvantages of the regime are that the tar preparation soils the clothes and sheets and is aesthetically displeasing because of the tar odour. This is why tar therapy is usually carried out only on an in-patient basis. However, the treatment is highly effective in the majority of patients, and the relapse rate is considerably lower than that of psoriasis treated with topical steroids.

### Dithranol

Dithranol is a highly effective therapeutic agent for chronic plaques of psoriasis on the limbs and trunk. It should not be used on the face, near the genitalia, or in the intertriginous areas.

It is advisable to begin treatment with a concentration of 0.1 per cent dithranol in Lassar's paste. The affected part of the body is then covered with tube-gauze dressings. The preparation should be applied daily to the lesions and then removed in a bath after 24 hours. If there is no significant improvement after a week and no untoward side effects then the concentration of the dithranol should be increased to 0.2 per cent and the concentration may be increased weekly up to 0.5 per cent if the lesions are slow to respond.

*Disadvantages of dithranol therapy.* Dithranol unfortunately stains the clothes and bed sheets a purplish colour, and thus lesions must be well protected by tube-gauze dressings. Dithranol also stains the normal skin surrounding the lesions a purplish-brown colour (Figure 8.31), and many patients find this embarrassing if the treated lesions are visible, e.g. hands and legs in women. Dithranol is also an irritant to the uninvolved skin. In its mildest form this irritation presents as erythema, but in some patients there is a severe reaction with blistering (Figure 8.32) and this will necessitate the discontinuation of dithranol treatment, or a significant reduction in the strength of dithranol used.

### Treatment of Psoriasis of the Scalp

Many of the preparations described above are unsuitable for psoriasis of the scalp, both for cosmetic reasons and because the condition is sometimes particularly resistant at this site. If the condition is mild then it may respond to topical steroids in a lotion or gel base specifically designed for use on the scalp. If the condition is more severe then a preparation containing tar and keratolytics will be required, e.g. 10 per cent coal tar solution B.P., 5 per cent sulphur, 5 per cent salicylic acid, 40 per cent coconut oil, 40 per cent emulsifying ointment B.P., which is a highly effective but rather 'messy' preparation. The patient however need not use such a preparation daily and if used weekly or twice weekly at night, with the preparation shampooed off the following morning, it may be sufficient to keep the condition under control.

### Systemic Treatment

#### Systemic Steroids

Systemic steroids play a very small part in the treatment of psoriasis. They should be used only if the above treatment regimes carried out in the wards have failed to control the condition. Systemic steroids have proved helpful in the past in generalised erythrodermic psoriasis. However, the problem with systemic steroids is that it is very difficult to wean the patients off the drug without a relapse of the psoriasis, and thus the problems and complications of long-term steroid therapy that may be encountered are probably not usually justified in the treatment of psoriasis.

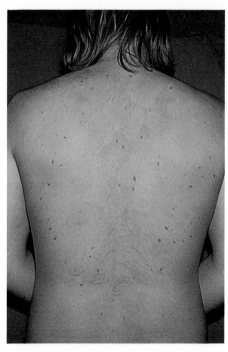

**Figure 8.33**
*Psoriasis beginning to clear due to PUVA treatment. The normal skin is beginning to tan.*

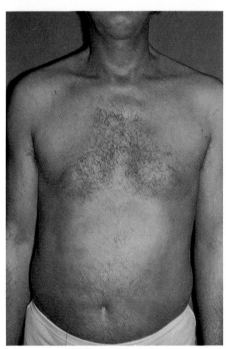

**Figure 8.34**
*Deep tan due to PUVA treatment. The psoriatic lesions have nearly disappeared, only residual erythema still being present. This will fade with further treatment.*

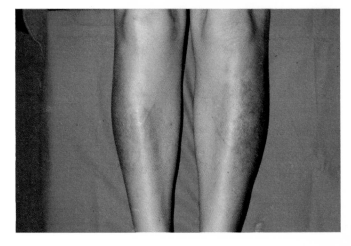

**Figure 8.35** (Right) *Localised areas of deeper pigmentation on the legs due to topical psoralens used in addition to systemic treatment.*

### Methotrexate

Methotrexate now appears to have some part to play in the management of severe and disabling psoriasis that cannot be controlled by other means. This drug should be given only under specialist supervision. The exact mechanism of action of methotrexate in psoriasis is unknown. It is thought that it may inhibit DNA synthesis which is increased in the epidermal cells in psoriasis. The advantage of methotrexate is that it may be given by mouth or intramuscular injection which patients with long-standing psoriasis find a relief after years of 'messy' ointments. However, methotrexate is a potentially dangerous drug with possible immediate damage to the bone-marrow and gastro-intestinal tract, long-term damage to the liver and even induction of malignancy.

### Photochemotherapy—PUVA

This is a relatively new approach to the problem of psoriasis. It has been known for many years that sunlight may help to clear psoriatic lesions. The drug psoralen (which occurs naturally in a plant, or may be synthesised) is a photo-sensitiser, increasing the effect of sunlight on the skin. It is the ultra-violet part of the spectrum which is beneficial in psoriasis. Ultra-violet light may be arbitrarily divided into short wave ultra-violet light 290–320 nm (known as UVB) and long wave ultra-violet light 320–400 nm (known as UVA). Short wave ultra-violet light, UVB, causes the reaction in the skin known as 'sunburn', whereas UVA does not have this damaging effect. However, in the presence of UVA, psoralen in the skin becomes chemically activated and enters into reactions, one of which is combination with DNA in the epidermal cells. Thus units containing lamps emitting UVA and no UVB have been designed for the treatment of psoriasis. Prior to irradiation with UVA the patients either took psoralen by mouth or used a topical psoralen preparation applied to the skin lesions. The ingestion or application of the psoralen must take place two hours before irradiation. It is thought that in the presence of UVA the psoralen combines with the DNA of the epidermal cells and blocks the 'psoriatic process'. This is at present speculation and not proven. The term PUVA is derived from P (for psoralen) + UVA.

The advantage of PUVA therapy is that it is effective when simpler measures have failed and that patients find it pleasant, for no messy ointments are required. The immediate disadvantage is that the treatment is time consuming. Patients need to attend on average four times a week for approximately one month. If the psoriasis is active then once or twice weekly maintenance therapy is required, because the relapse rate in active psoriasis is high. The possible long-term side effects have still to be evaluated.

One of the effects of PUVA treatment is a deep tan (Figures 8.33, 8.34 and 8.35) which develops during treatment. This is due to the effect of UVA and psoralen on the melanocytes. Most patients find the tan pleasing and it eventually fades if treatment is stopped.

### General Measures

*Diet.* Patients often ask whether they should miss out any particular food or have any extra vitamins or minerals in their diet. At the present time there is no evidence that any dietary restrictions or additions make any difference to psoriasis.

*Sunlight.* Natural sunlight frequently helps psoriasis, but it can also make it worse, particularly if the patients over expose themselves and become 'burnt'. Patients should be warned of this. It is interesting that near the Dead Sea, where there is a unit for the treatment of psoriasis, the UVB of the sunlight is screened out by the aerosol effect of the water vapour rising from the sea. This effect is unique to the climatic and geographic conditions of the area.

*Psychiatric treatment.* There is no good evidence that patients with psoriasis are basically more neurotic than controls without psoriasis. However, it is not surprising that many patients with such a disfiguring condition may become depressed. But it must be admitted that in certain individuals emotional problems will precipitate or aggravate the condition, and these problems should be dealt with by the appropriate means.

*Psoriasis Association.* Recently a 'Psoriasis Association' has been founded in Great Britain and one of its aims is to help sufferers with this condition. It is well worthwhile for patients with psoriasis to be put in touch with this society if their disorder is causing social problems.

# 9. Pityriasis Rosea and Lichen Planus

## Pityriasis Rosea

PITYRIASIS rosea is one of the so-called papulosquamous eruptions. The term pityriasis is derived from a Greek word meaning 'branlike'. Pityriasis rosea is a common dermatosis of unknown aetiology, but with characteristic lesions and a good prognosis. The disorder tends to affect males and females equally. It is rare in infancy and old age, and affects mainly young adults. It occurs more commonly in a temperate climate and appears predominantly in the spring and autumn.

Pityriasis rosea usually begins with a solitary lesion, 'the herald patch' (Figure 9.1). This lesion is nearly always on the trunk, and never on the face. The lesion is an annular scaly patch, with a slightly raised edge, and is reddish-brown in colour. At this stage the lesion may be mistaken for tinea corporis. On direct questioning the patient may admit a mild sore throat and malaise. Within one to two weeks other lesions, which are usually smaller than the herald patch, begin to appear on the trunk. The lesions occur mostly on the trunk (Figure 9.2), but may also involve the neck and upper parts of the limbs; the face, hands and feet are only very rarely affected. The lesions tend to be oval with their long axes in the lines of cleavage of the skin (Figures 9.3 and 9.4). Another characteristic and diagnostically helpful feature of the lesions that may be visible is centripetal scaling (Figures 9.5 and 9.6). Occasionally they may have a different appearance and present as small papules 3–4 mm in diameter with a slightly scaly surface. This is sometimes referred to as papular pityriasis rosea.

The severity of pityriasis rosea varies a great deal; the lesions may be so numerous that practically all of the skin of the trunk is affected (Figure 9.6), or there may be only a few scattered on the limbs and trunk (Figure 9.3). Apart from the appearances the disease is frequently symptomless, although sometimes there is occasional irritation. The disorder runs a self-limiting course and clears within two to three months of onset.

It is extremely uncommon for patients to develop a further attack of pityriasis rosea and because of this an infectious aetiology with subsequent immunity has been suggested, but this has not been proved.

The differential diagnosis of pityriasis rosea includes secondary syphilis, some forms of eczema, psoriasis, and tinea corporis.

### Treatment

Once the patient has been reassured as to the benign nature of the condition and the fact that the disorder has a self-limiting course, no active treatment is usually required. Suppression or partial suppression of the lesions may be obtained with intermediate strength corticosteroid prepara-

**Figure 9.2** *Oval and discoid red lesions on the trunk in pityriasis rosea.*

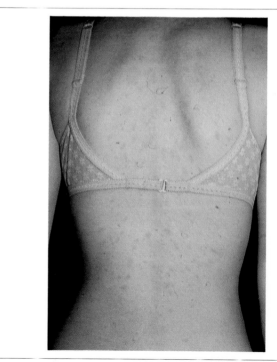

**Figure 9.1** *Herald patch in pityriasis rosea. The lesion is often annular and larger than the other lesions.*

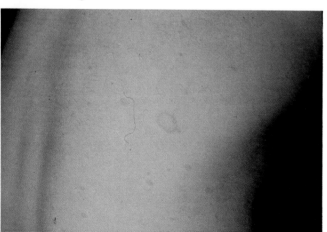

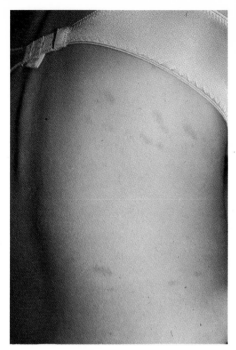

**Figure 9.3** *Pityriasis rosea. Oval lesions on the side of the trunk. The long axes are in the direction of the lines of cleavage of the skin.*

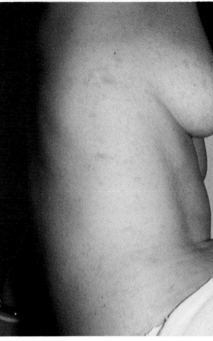

**Figure 9.4** *Pityriasis rosea. Lesions of varying size, those lesions which are oval have their long axes in the lines of cleavage of the skin.*

**Figure 9.5** *Lesion of pityriasis rosea showing centri-petal scaling.*

tions. If there is any associated irritation, then topical corticosteroids as described above should be used twice daily and systemic antihistamines, such as trimeprazine 10 mg t.d.s., should be prescribed.

### Lichen Planus

Lichen planus is another of the papulosquamous eruptions of unknown aetiology. It is not as common a dermatosis as psoriasis, but it does account for one per cent of all new cases seen in a skin clinic, compared to five per cent for psoriasis.

The term lichen planus means a flat topped papule, and this is the commonest form of presentation of the disorder. Lichen planus affects mainly young and middle-aged adults, and males and females are equally affected.

#### Morphology and Distribution

The appearances of the lesions vary with the site of involvement. The commonest and most typical lesion is the flat topped papule which often has a 'shiny' surface (Figures 9.7 and 9.8). The lesions are usually small, approximately 5 mm in diameter. They are either red or have a violaceous colour (Figure 9.9), and occasionally white streaks (Wickham's striae) can be seen on the surface of the lesions (Figures 9.8 and 9.10). There may be slight central umbilication of the lesion. The papules may affect any part of the skin, but the commonest site is the wrists (Figure 9.11). The severity of the disease may vary from the presence of a few scattered papules to the whole skin being covered with numerous papules.

Occasionally the lesions fuse to form plaques (Figure 9.9), which have a similar violaceous colour, and white streaks

**Figure 9.6** *A more acute form of pityriasis rosea with widespread involvement. A number of lesions show centri-petal scaling.*

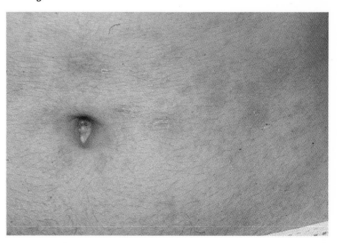

may still be discernible. Lichen planus, like psoriasis, shows the Koebner phenomenon, i.e. the lesions will appear in a linear pattern along a scratch mark or any kind of trauma to the skin.

Lichen planus on the legs and occasionally on the arms may take the form of what is termed 'hypertrophic lichen planus' (Figures 9.12 and 9.13). In this instance the lesions are plaque-like and have a thick warty (hyperkeratotic) surface. This type of lichen planus may be difficult to distinguish from patches of chronic eczema if there are no classical lesions of lichen planus at other sites. In very acute cases of lichen planus the lesions may form blisters (Figure 9.14).

47

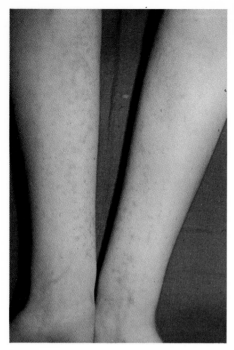

**Figure 9.7** *Papules of lichen planus on the forearms, some with a 'shiny' surface.*

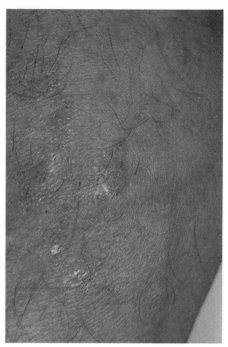

**Figure 9.8** *Lichen planus. The lesions have a shiny surface and white streaks (Wickham's striae) are visible in the largest lesion.*

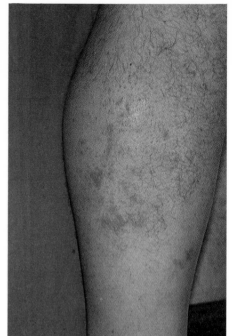

**Figure 9.9** *Violaceous lesions of lichen planus on the leg. There is a tendency to plaque formation.*

**Figure 9.10** *White streaks (Wickham's striae) in lichen planus.*

**Figure 9.11** *The wrists are amongst the commonest sites for lichen planus.*

**Figure 9.12** *Plaque of hypertrophic lichen planus. The leg is the commonest site for this form of lichen planus.*

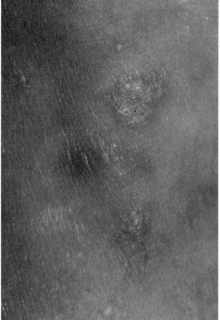

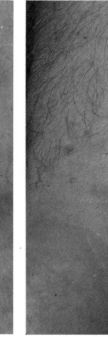

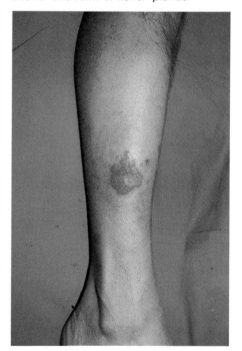

Lichen planus is associated with increased pigmentation, and when the lesions clear there is often residual hyperpigmentation for many weeks or months. In coloured persons lichen planus presents as hyperpigmented papules (Figure 9.15).

*Scalp*—this is not a common site of involvement, but the important fact is that on the scalp lichen planus may produce atrophy of the skin with subsequent loss of hair (Figure 9.16). The hair loss tends to be patchy, but is permanent.

*Nails*—the disease process can also affect the nail matrix. Usually the involvement of the nails is minimal and presents as longitudinal ridging which eventually clears. Occasionally there is severe involvement of the nails with pterygium formation (the cuticle grows forward and

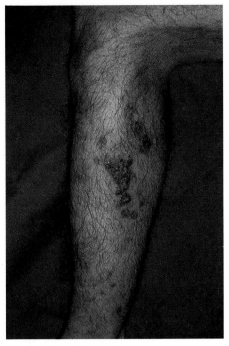

**Figure 9.13** *Warty hyperpigmented lesions of hypertrophic lichen planus.*

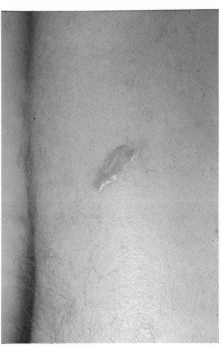

**Figure 9.14** *Blister formation which may occur in a lichen planus lesion.*

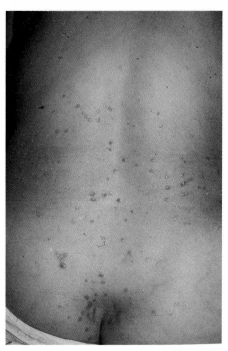

**Figure 9.15** *Lichen planus presenting as hyperpigmented papules in a dark skinned person. Hyperpigmentation is common in lichen planus.*

**Figure 9.16**
*Patchy hair loss following lichen planus of the scalp.*

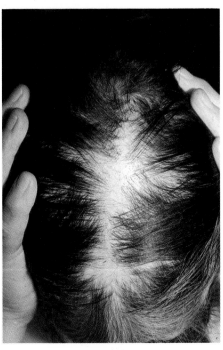

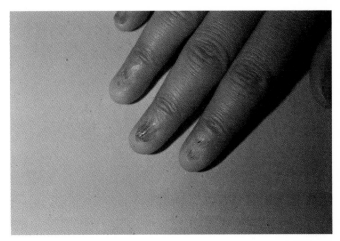

**Figure 9.17** *Lichen planus of the nails. Severe involvement with pterygium formation and permanent loss of the nail plate on some fingers.*

attaches itself to the nail plate), and there may be permanent loss of the nail plate (Figure 9.17).

*Palms and soles*—because of the thick keratin at these sites, the appearances of the disorder are modified. Although the lesions may present as small papules, they do not have the flat topped appearance with white streaks but often present as hyperkeratotic brownish papules. If the lesions merge to-gether, hyperkeratotic plaques (Figure 9.18) are formed which become fissured, and the appearances are then similar to psoriasis at this site or to chronic eczema.

*Mucous membranes and genitalia*—the buccal mucosa is the commonest site of involvement (with lesions at other sites in about 50 per cent of cases). In the early stages there are small white papules which subsequently fuse to form a white lace pattern (Figure 9.19). It is important to remember to examine the buccal mucosa when lichen planus is suspected from lesions on the skin; if it is involved it will establish the diagnosis. The lips, gums and tongue (Figure 9.20) may also be similarly affected, as may be the vulval and vaginal

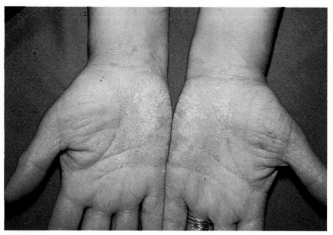

**Figure 9.18** *Hyperkeratotic plaques on the palms due to lichen planus. The typical papules are seen on the wrists.*

**Figure 9.19** *Lichen planus of the buccal mucosa with white papules and streaks.*

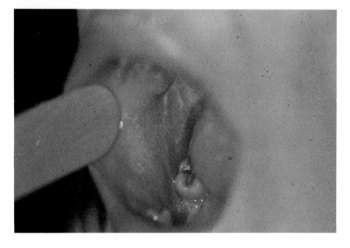

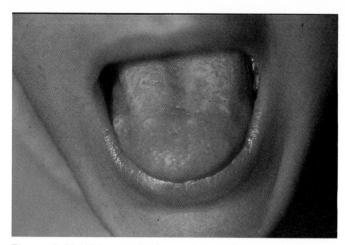

**Figure 9.20** *White streaks, becoming confluent in some areas, in lichen planus of the tongue.*

**Figure 9.21** *Annular white lesions on the glans penis in lichen planus.*

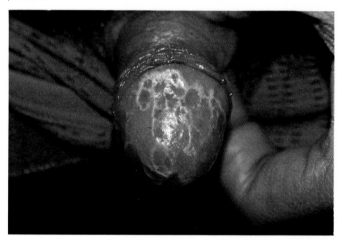

**Figure 9.22** *Lichen planus of the tongue. White patches and erosions.*

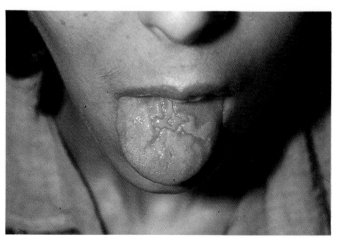

mucosa. On the glans penis the white streaks often join to form annular lesions (Figure 9.21). Occasionally only the oral cavity and genitalia are involved. There are reports of lichen planus of the mucosal surfaces progressing to leukoplakia and even carcinoma, but this is a very rare complication. The vast majority of the lesions at these sites will undergo spontaneous resolution.

### Erosive Lichen Planus

Occasionally the lesions on the mucosal surfaces, particularly the gums and tongue (Figure 9.22), may present as erosions rather than the white plaque-like lesions.

### Duration and Recurrence

If untreated, lichen planus usually lasts for several months and then tends to disappear. The hypertrophic forms of the disorder tend to be persistent and may last for many years. Similarly, erosive lichen planus of the mouth and genitalia tends to be persistent. Approximately 20 per cent of patients will have a relapse of the condition after a first episode.

### Aetiology

The cause of lichen planus is unknown, and although a viral or other infective agent has been considered, these hypotheses, have not been confirmed. A number of drugs, notably mepacrine, chloroquin, gold and para-amino-salicylic acid, may induce an eruption which clinically may be indistinguishable from lichen planus.

## Treatment

If the condition consists of only a few lesions, no treatment may be required. However, the lesions are frequently associated with irritation and this in itself often leads to the patient seeking help. Intermediate strength topical corticosteroid preparations are helpful in alleviating the irritation and appear to be able to induce a clearance of the lesions in some instances. If there is no significant response to the intermediate strength steroids, then a short course, i.e. two to three weeks, of a strong topical steroid should be given and this may suppress the lesions. If, however, the disease is very widespread, then systemic corticosteroids are probably justified and are certainly a more acceptable form of treatment as far as the patient is concerned. A dose of prednisone 30 mg daily will probably be required for at least two weeks, and then the dose may be reduced gradually over the next two weeks. The majority of patients will remain free after treatment, but 20–25 per cent will have a recurrence of the disorder. The lesions on the mucous membranes usually require no treatment, particularly if confined to the buccal mucosa. However, if they are severe and are causing discomfort, they may respond to corticosteroid mouth lozenges or aerosols, and betamethasone 17-valerate lozenges have recently been found to be effective for resistant cases. Occasionally systemic steroids as a long-term measure are required for the severe and erosive forms of lichen planus.

The hypertrophic forms of lichen planus on the limbs respond well to intralesional injections of triamcinolone.

# 10. Fungal Infections

DISORDERS of the skin, hair and nails caused by fungus are still common in dermatological practice, and the importance of establishing the correct diagnosis has become greater over the last decade for two reasons. First, with the discovery and clinical application of the anti-fungal griseofulvin there is now an effective agent for successfully treating a large number of fungus infections of the skin, nails and hair. Second, the powerful topical corticosteroids are used to treat many fungal infections because the disease has been incorrectly diagnosed or just considered to be another 'rash' which will clear with this modern panacea. Unless this is realised these disorders which are easily treatable become unnecessarily chronic and troublesome complaints.

There are many thousands of species of fungi, but like bacteria only a minority are pathogenic to the human. These may be arbitrarily divided into those affecting the skin and those capable of deep invasion and causing systemic disease. However, a few species, such as monilia, may affect the skin and also cause systemic disease.

The fungi causing skin disease generally live in keratin and do not affect the deeper and viable parts of the skin. However, possibly when the immune mechanisms of the host are upset, fungi do rarely invade the dermis with the production of abscesses or granulomatous nodules.

## Ringworm

This is a lay term for fungus infections, which has arisen because a number of fungus infections of the skin begin as small inflammatory lesions but subsequently spread out to form annular or ring lesions. The disorders the fungus cause are referred to as tineas (from the latin word 'tinea' meaning a 'gnawing worm') usually with the qualifying noun depending on the part of the body affected, e.g. tinea capitis. The fungus actually lives in the keratin, producing enzymes which break the keratin, thus giving rise to a clinical lesion affecting the skin, hair or nails.

There are three genera of ringworm fungi: Trichophyton, Microsporum and Epidermophyton. A few of these species produce characteristic lesions at certain sites of the body but often the clinical manifestations of the different species are similar, and require culture for specific mycological diagnosis. Some species of fungi are pathogenic only to humans while others are pathogenic to animals and humans. The species which affect only humans produce persistent non-inflammatory lesions whereas ringworm contracted from animals tends to be inflammatory and shortlived.

Ringworm infections, although contagious, are not as infectious as is generally believed by the lay public. It seems that many subjects, although repeatedly exposed to ringworm fungi—such as in a family where one member is affected—have keratin with properties which do not permit the fungus to grow and produce clinical lesions.

### Diagnosis

Examining scrapings of the skin, or specimens of nail and hair in 10 per cent potassium hydroxide is an easy and simple way of establishing the diagnosis. The potassium

**Figure 10.1** *Demonstration of fungal hyphae in keratin. Skin scrapings have been soaked in 10 per cent potassium hydroxide for 20 minutes and the hyphae are now easily seen on microscopy.*

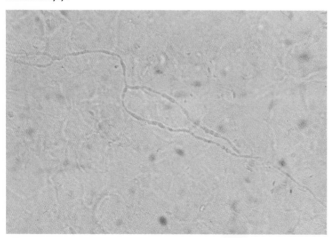

**Figure 10.2** *Scaling and erythema on the sides of the toes, the commonest site for a fungal infection.*

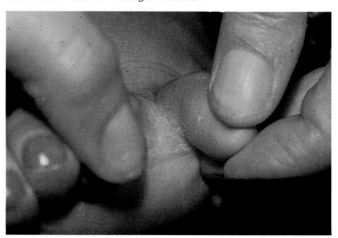

hydroxide dissolves the keratin and the fungi are then easily seen by microscopy (Figure 10.1). The alternative or additional method is to culture the infected keratin in Sabouraud's medium. However, although this is necessary to establish the species, it takes two to three weeks for the fungus to grow and with the advent of griseofulvin, which affects the majority of superficial ringworm species, culturing will not usually be required in the clinical management of the disorder.

## Management

*Griseofulvin* is an anti-fungal agent which has radically altered the management of superficial fungus infections. It has to be given by mouth to be effective, and has to be deposited in the keratin to eradicate the fungus. This mechanism of action has to be appreciated, so that the length of time for which the drug has to be given will depend on the site of the keratin affected by the fungus. The epidermis (which has no blood vessels) takes approximately one month to 'replace itself'. The basal cells in the lower part of the epidermis have the griseofulvin deposited in them within 24 hours of taking the drug by mouth and it takes a month for these cells to move upwards and replace the keratin which is affected by the fungus. Similarly, when treating fungus infections of the hair and nails the length of time required for the new 'griseofulvin impregnated' hair or nails to grow has to be appreciated. Griseofulvin does not penetrate into infected dead keratinous structures, but is deposited only as new keratin is formed.

*Side effects of griseofulvin.* Fortunately these are very few and rare, and griseofulvin is probably one of the antibiotics with the lowest incidence of side effects. The commonest problem encountered is gastrointestinal upset, usually nausea. Headaches and drug rashes have been recorded, the latter taking the form of urticaria or morbilliform eruption. It may have some slight adverse effect on liver function and it may affect the prothrombin time in patients on anticoagulants, although, provided this is appreciated, it is in itself no contraindication to the use of the drug.

*Topical anti-fungal preparations.* There are numerous topical anti-fungal preparations available for treatment of fungal infections of the skin. However, in the clinical situation, none are 100 per cent effective. It is probably best to become accustomed to one or two topical preparations and to use only those. In most instances Whitfield's ointment B.P. (6 per cent benzoic acid and 3 per cent salicylic acid) is as effective as the newer preparations and is considerably cheaper. Miconazole nitrate and clotrimazole are two of the newer preparations used in cream bases for ringworm infections of the skin. They are expensive and do not appear to have any advantage over Whitfield's ointment other than being more pleasant to use.

## Ringworm of the Feet (Tinea Pedis)

The feet are the commonest site for fungal infections. This is probably due to the fact that fungus grows better in moist rather than dry areas, and the close fit of the toes and footwear fashions are both contributory factors in encouraging the growth of fungus.

Fungal infection of the feet tends to be a disease of young and middle-aged adults, and is commoner in males than females. It is rare in children. The exact mode of transmission is not certain and although swimming pools, showers etc., are implicated as the usual source, host susceptibility is obviously an important factor for familial cross-infections are rarely seen.

### Clinical Presentation

In the majority of patients tinea pedis is manifested by peeling and slight maceration of the skin between the toes (Figure 10.2). The peeling usually extends onto the plantar surface of the toes, and this clinical point is useful in distinguishing tinea pedis from eczema or psoriasis between the toes (Figure 10.3). The peeling and scaling may involve any of the interdigital spaces although it is very rarely seen between the first and second toes. The disorder is frequently confined to the interdigital spaces and gives rise only to slight irritation. However, the disease may become more extensive and involve the sole. If the infecting fungus is Tinea

**Figure 10.3** *Scaling extending on to the surface of the toes in a fungal infection. This helps to distinguish the condition from eczema and psoriasis.*

**Figure 10.4** *Acute exudative eruption occasionally seen in fungal infections of the feet.*

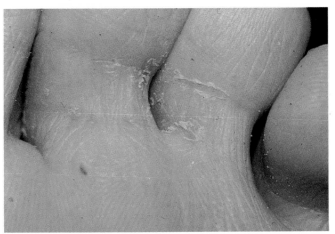

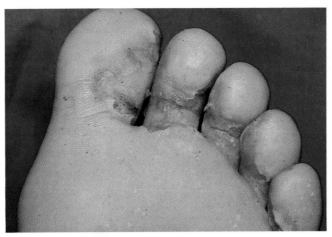

rubrum then the disease is manifested as diffuse scaling and hyperkeratosis. If the organism is T. mentagrophytes then the disorder may be represented by blisters and acute exudative dermatitis (Figure 10.4), either on the soles or extending from the interdigital spaces on to the dorsum of the foot.

### Differential Diagnosis

It is important that not all scaly skin between and around the toes is attributed to fungus, as other conditions can also cause this appearance and the treatment is different. Simple maceration of the skin due to excess sweating is probably the commonest differential diagnosis but psoriasis and eczema may also affect only the distal half of the foot.

### Treatment

Unfortunately, griseofulvin has not resulted in eradication of the fungus and cure of the disorder when it affects the feet. However, if griseofulvin is given for a month in the normal dose of 500 mg daily the skin will become normal but the relapse rate is so high and rapid that griseofulvin is not indicated if the disorder is confined simply to the interdigital spaces. In these instances topical anti-fungal agents should be used and Whitfield's ointment B.P. (benzoic acid and salicylic acid) is still clinically the most effective. If the skin is macerated it is often helpful to apply pig. magenta once a day to keep the skin dry. General advice on drying well between the toes after bathing, and the use of ventilated footwear, if possible, is important.

In an extensive T. rubrum infection with scaling on the soles of the feet, griseofulvin is indicated in a dose of 500 mg daily for four to six weeks. The relapse rate for the more general involvement of the sole of the foot is considerably lower than that for the interdigital spaces.

### Acute Inflammatory Fungal Infections of the Feet

These should be treated like an eczema in the early stages. Potassium permanganate soaks 1:8,000 q.d.s. for 10 minutes on each occasion and clean linen dressings should be used. One per cent hydrocortisone lotion may help to settle the inflammation. As it settles, the irritation may be relieved by 1 per cent hydrocortisone cream. The condition may subside with these simple measures. Griseofulvin has no part to play in the acute stages because of its mode of action, but it should be given to prevent an immediate relapse, particularly in warm weather.

### Ringworm of the Hands

This is very much rarer than that of the feet. It is usually caused by T. rubrum and presents as a slight erythema and diffuse scaling of the palmar surface of the hands (Figure 10.5). The diagnosis should be established by demonstrating the fungus and treatment is with griseofulvin 500 mg daily for four weeks.

### Ringworm of the Groins (Tinea Cruris)

This is the second commonest site to be involved after the feet. It is commoner in males than females. The infection usually begins in the crural fold as erythema and slight maceration. It spreads out in an annular pattern with a raised red scaly margin (Figure 10.6). It may spread down the thigh or sometimes backwards up to the buttock. The disorder in the early stages has to be distinguished from intertrigo (seborrhoeic eczema) and intertriginous psoriasis.

**Figure 10.5** *Diffuse scaling and erythema on the palmar surface of the hand due to T. rubrum infection.*

**Figure 10.6** *Tinea cruris. The eruption spreads from the groins on to the thighs, and often has a raised, scaly edge.*

**Figure 10.7** *A typical annular ringworm lesion.*

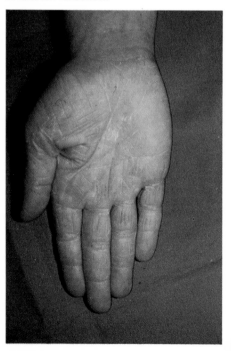

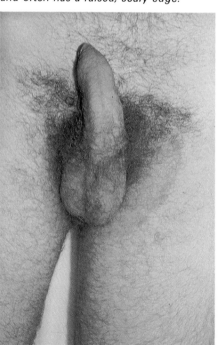

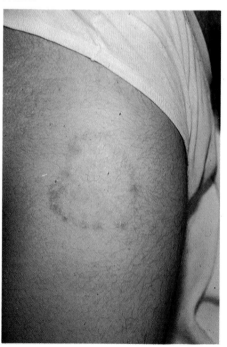

### Treatment

As much aeration as possible is important to allow evaporation of perspiration in this area and thus tight-fitting undergarments should be avoided. If there is acute inflammation, then sitz baths with potassium permanganate solution 1:8,000, or daily application of magenta paint will be helpful. One per cent hydrocortisone lotion should be used two or three times a day to decrease inflammation. In the more common presentation with chronic, red, scaly lesions, griseofulvin 500 mg daily for a month should be prescribed. Topical anti-fungal preparations may be tried if the eruption is minimal and confined to the groins. Relapse of fungus infections in the groins is fairly frequent, and conditions leading to excess moisture should be avoided if possible.

### Ringworm of the Body (Tinea Corporis)

*Annular lesions.* This is the characteristic type of lesion which even lay people are familiar with as being due to a fungus. The lesion usually begins as a small red papule and then advances to form a ring (Figure 10.7). Occasionally, however, there is no clearing in the centre and an oval or discoid red scaly plaque is the presenting feature (Figure 10.8). Treatment is with griseofulvin 125 mg t.d.s in children and 500 mg daily in adults.

*Tinea granuloma.* This may take one of two forms. It can be a discrete infiltrating granuloma of the skin which will have to be distinguished from other skin granulomata (Figure 10.9). This type of lesion is usually caused by a fungus from an animal source. Although the lesions are usually self-involuting, griseofulvin 500 mg daily should be given for four to six weeks. The other type of granuloma is found on the hairy parts of the limbs, for it is an infection around the hair follicles and there are often small papules (Figure 10.10) and pustules present. The diagnosis is frequently missed. It should be thought of if there is a chronic unilateral inflammatory process on an arm or leg. The disorder responds well to a month's course of griseofulvin.

### Ringworm of the Scalp (Tinea Capitis)

Tinea capitis is due to fungus affecting the hair (which is a form of keratin) and the skin keratin of the scalp.

The fungal infections of the scalp due to organisms which cause fluorescence of the hairs with ultra-violet irradiation, 330–360 nm (Wood's Light), are confined almost entirely to children. Non-fluorescent ringworm of the scalp occurs both in children and adults. The fungi which cause fluorescence are *Microsporum audouini* and *Microsporum canis,* the latter being derived from animals, usually cats. The commonest organism to cause ringworm of the scalp is *Microsporum audouini.* The condition is contagious and minor epidemics may often be found in schools.

### Clinical Features

The disease usually presents as a small oval or discoid patch on any part of the scalp. The predominant feature is loss of hair (Figure 10.11). If the lesion is carefully examined it will be seen that the hairs are broken off near to the skin surface and there is not complete or uniform loss of hair. The skin is usually scaly and nearly always affected in addition to the hair keratin (Figures 10.12 and 10.13). These two features of a scaly base, and broken hairs at varying lengths as opposed to complete loss of hair are important physical signs in distinguishing the condition from alopecia areata

**Figure 10.8** *Discoid, red, scaly lesion due to a fungal infection on the trunk.*

**Figure 10.9** *Granuloma on the forearm due to a fungal infection.*

**Figure 10.10** *Granulomatous fungal infection of the back of the hand and forearm. Small papules are present around the hair follicles.*

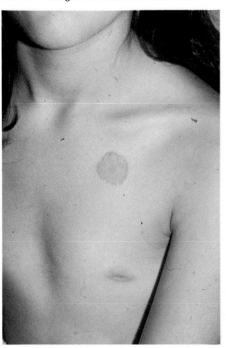

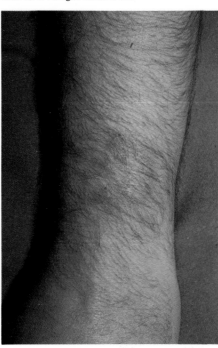

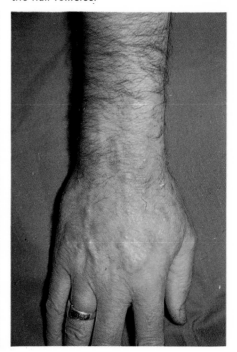

(although occasionally in the latter there may not be complete baldness but a diffuse loss). Involvement of the scalp with fungus may occur as a solitary lesion or multiple lesions (Figure 10.13) with sometimes nearly the whole of the scalp involved. In addition to the scalp lesions there are often scaly discoid patches on the neck just below the hair-line.

As the infection with the fungus persists signs of inflammation will appear. Apart from the skin being scaly, erythema and pustules develop (Figure 10.14). If there is progression of the inflammation then the whole of the area shows signs of an acute inflammatory process with swelling, redness of the tissues, pustule formation, and occasionally superficial ulceration. This type of lesion is known as a kerion. It is thought to be due to the tissues developing an inflammatory immune response to the fungi, and, therefore, is ultimately self-healing. Despite the rather alarming appearance it will eventually subside even without specific treatment and does not lead to scarring and permanent hair loss. Tinea capitis due to the fungus contracted from animals (*M. canis*) tends to produce an inflammatory response more frequently than that caused by *M. audouini*.

The fungi which may affect the hair and scalp keratin, but do not cause fluorescence of the hairs with ultra-violet irradiation, do not always produce the same classical clinical appearances as those caused by the *M. audouini* and *M. canis*. Usually the only constant sign is the hairs breaking off at the scalp surface producing an area of 'black dots'. This type of lesion will have to be distinguished from the hair being broken due to trauma (trichotillomania) in which the hairs are not usually broken so close to the surface of the scalp. If there are associated inflammatory changes the condition has to be distinguished from excoriated seborrhoeic eczema or psoriasis.

### Diagnosis

The diagnosis of tinea capitis depends on the demonstration of the fungus. In the disorder due to *M. audouini* or *M. canis* this can be simply done by Wood's light examination, the affected hairs showing a green fluorescence. Ideally, specimens of the hair and scale from the scalp surface should also be taken for microscopical examination and cultured to confirm the diagnosis. In cases of non-fluorescent tinea capitis, the diagnosis has to be made by microscopy of the hair and scales and subsequent culture.

If a child of school age has tinea capitis it is the usual practice to screen other children who come into contact

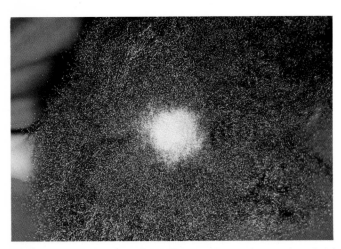

**Figure 10.11** *Tinea capitis. The presenting feature is a bald patch.*

**Figure 10.12** *Scaling of the skin as well as hair loss is present in tinea capitis, distinguishing it from alopecia areata.*

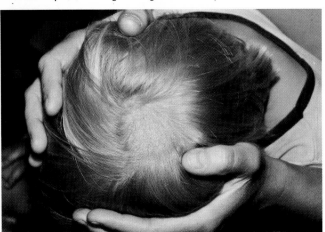

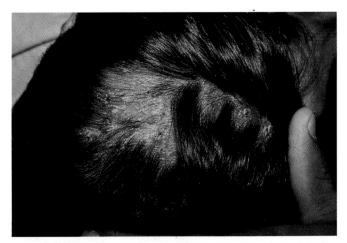

**Figure 10.13** *Multiple areas of the scalp affected by a fungal infection. The surface is usually scaly and the hair loss is not complete.*

**Figure 10.14** *Inflammatory changes, erythema and pustules, in tinea capitis.*

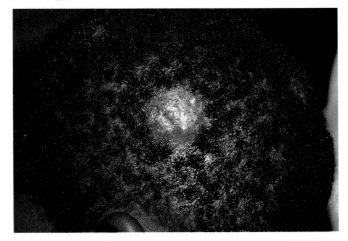

with him at school. Since the majority of the cases are due to fungi which cause the hairs to fluoresce, the screening can be done by Wood's light examination. Other methods that are now employed and reported as giving a higher incidence of positive pick-up include brushing the hair thoroughly and subsequently putting the brush under a Wood's light, or placing the brush in a plate of culture medium and seeing if there is subsequent growth of the fungus.

All children who have tinea capitis will have to be kept away from school until they are clear of fungus, judged by the clinical appearance and Wood's light examination (if positive in the first instance).

### Treatment

With the advent of griseofulvin the management of tinea capitis has been revolutionised. At least one month's treatment with griseofulvin 125 mg t.d.s. will be required. The new hair which will be impregnated with griseofulvin and, therefore, free of fungus takes three to four weeks to grow out of the hair follicle. After two to three weeks of therapy it is advisable to clip the hair surrounding the lesions to remove the fungi remaining in the distal part of the hair.

It is sometimes difficult to persuade young children to take tablets and in these instances griseofulvin suspension should be prescribed. The dose is the same as for the tablet form of the drug.

If there is no satisfactory response it may mean the child is not taking the griseofulvin, or is taking another drug such as phenobarbitone which may interfere with the metabolism of griseofulvin. In the former instance one large dose of griseofulvin, e.g. 2 g weekly taken under supervision of the doctor or nursing staff may be satisfactory in producing a cure.

### Ringworm of the Nails (Tinea Unguium)

Both the toe- and finger-nails can be involved although the toe-nails are more commonly affected. The disorder may be caused by species of Trichophyton and Epidermophyton but not Microsporum.

### Clinical Features

Ringworm fungi usually begin to invade the nail by first affecting the lateral nail grooves where there is soft keratin. The infection then spreads into the lateral portions of the nail plate, and usually causes a yellowish discoloration (Figure 10.15). Infection then usually spreads to involve the nail-bed and may cause considerable hyperkeratosis (Figures 10.16 and 10.17). The process may stop at any stage or may continue subsequently to involve the whole of the nail-bed and nail-plate, although the nail matrix is not affected. Apart from the subungual hyperkeratosis, involvement of the nail-plate may produce considerable distortion of this structure (Figure 10.18).

Ringworm of the nails usually involves only one or two nails initially, and this may be confined to one hand or foot. The involvement of the nails in a hand or foot is often variable (Figure 10.19), unlike psoriasis in which the dystrophy

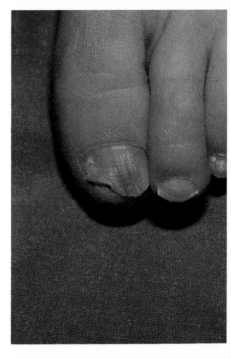

**Figure 10.15**
*Yellowish discoloration of the nail due to a fungal infection. The infection begins at the side and spreads across the nail.*

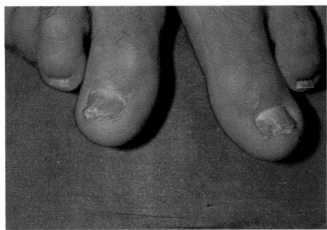

**Figure 10.16**
(Below)
*Subungual hyperkeratosis of the toe nails due to a fungal infection.*

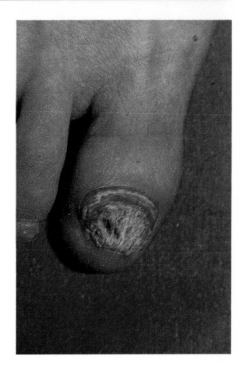

**Figure 10.17**
*Severe deformity and thickening due to a chronic fungal infection of the nail.*

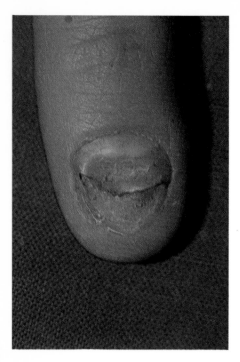

**Figure 10.18**
*Deformity of a finger nail due to a fungal infection.*

the latter presents as subungual hyperkeratosis. Dystrophy of the nails caused by monilia (*Candida albicans*) is often diagnosed prior to hospital attendance as being a ringworm infection. The important distinguishing factor is that with a monilial infection there is a chronic paronychia and with ringworm fungus the nail-fold usually has a normal appearance. Both eczema and lichen planus may cause nail dystrophies by involvement of the nail matrix in the disease process. It is important to realise that diseases other than ringworm can cause dystrophies which on clinical grounds may sometimes be difficult to diagnose. Thus before embarking on treatment for ringworm of the nails, it is very important that the diagnosis has been established by demonstrating the presence of the fungus.

### Treatment

Ringworm infection of the finger-nails usually responds well to treatment with griseofulvin. However, since a finger-nail may take up to six months to replace itself completely this is the length of time for which griseofulvin, 500 mg daily, will have to be given. Usually there is a good response and a very high cure rate for finger-nail infection. Infection of toe-nails, however, does not respond so well. The reasons for the poor response are not completely understood, but one reason sometimes put forward is that toe-nails infected by ringworm do not grow normally, and therefore the fungus cannot be eradicated. If treatment with griseofulvin is decided upon for toe-nail infection it may have to be given for up to two years to result in a cure and the relapse rate on cessation of treatment is high. If only one or two toe-nails are affected some authorities advise removal of the nail-plate after a month's course of griseofulvin and continuation of the griseofulvin until the new nail has grown. However, since the results of treatment of toe-nail infection are poor and the relapse rate high some dermatologists do not consider it worthwhile to treat toe-nail infection with griseofulvin. Each case should be considered individually and the possible reasons for treatment considered. Women often want treatment for cosmetic reasons, and occasionally the dystrophic nail causes discomfort.

tends to be uniform. Subsequently other nails may become involved until all the nails of both feet or hands are affected (Figure 10.20). Why the nails are affected by fungi in some persons who have skin involvement (particularly feet), but not in others is unknown. Many persons have ringworm infection between the toes for many years and never have involvement of the nails.

### Diagnosis

Since any treatment undertaken will be continued for a considerable length of time it is important to establish the correct diagnosis before commencing therapy. Specimens of the affected nail-plate and the hyperkeratotic material from the nail-bed should be examined by microscopy and culture for fungus.

The most common differential diagnosis of a fungal infection of the nails is probably psoriasis, particularly when

**Figure 10.19** *Asymmetrical involvement of the nails in a fungal infection.*

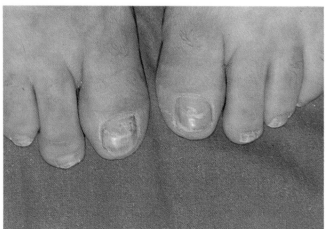

**Figure 10.20** *Long-standing fungal infection of the finger nails. All the nails are affected but to varying degrees.*

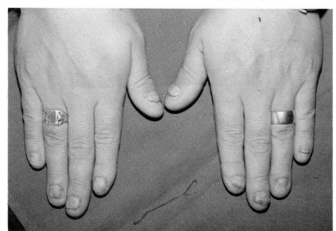

## Tinea Versicolor

This condition is also sometimes known as pityriasis versicolor. The word versicolor means change of colour and is a very apt description of the disorder. Tinea versicolor is caused by a fungus, *Malassezia furfur*, which affects only the stratum corneum.

### Clinical Features

The typical lesion of pityriasis versicolor is a fawn coloured macular patch of varying shape and size (Figure 10.21), but often patches may coalesce to form confluent areas on the upper trunk (Figure 10.22). The surface is sometimes scaly and scale can easily be produced from a lesion by gently scraping with a scalpel. If the patient exposes himself to sunlight then the areas of the skin affected by the fungus do *not* pigment, and they appear as white patches against a tanned skin (Figure 10.23). This is frequently the presenting manifestation after the patient has been on holiday.

The commonest site to be affected is the upper trunk although the neck and upper arms may also be involved.

### Diagnosis

The diagnosis is easily made on clinical grounds alone, but can be confirmed by examining skin scrapings by microscopy after dissolving the keratin with 10 per cent potassium hydroxide. The microscopic appearance is diagnostic. The hyphae are short and numerous clusters of spores are seen.

### Treatment

Pityriasis versicolor does not respond to griseofulvin. Topical applications have to be used and they are effective, but unfortunately there is a high incidence of recurrence. The topical applications which may be used are the shampoo Selenium Sulphide (Selsun), half-strength Whitfield's Ointment B.N.P., or 25 per cent aqueous solution of sodium thiosulphate. Treatment will have to be carried out daily for three to four weeks. There is no indication for using the newer and more expensive topical antifungal preparations.

## Erythrasma

This is usually considered with fungal diseases, although the causative organism has now been shown to be a bacterium, *Corynebacterium minutissimum*.

### Clinical Features

The areas affected are intertriginous, namely groins, axillae, between the toes, and under the breasts. The lesions are confluent, reddish-brown, scaly patches. There is no associated inflammation which tends to distinguish the condition from seborrhoeic eczema. Under Wood's light there is a pink fluorescence, which helps in establishing the diagnosis. There have been reports that erythrasma may be

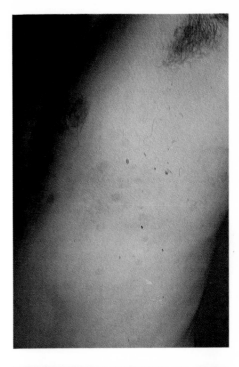

**Figure 10.21**
*Typical light-brown, slightly scaly lesions of pityriasis versicolor.*

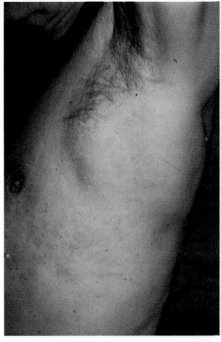

**Figure 10.22**
*Extensive pityriasis versicolor, the lesions becoming confluent.*

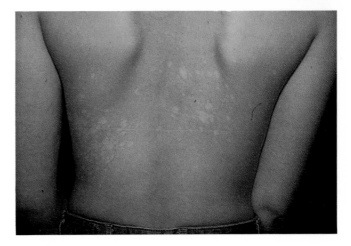

**Figure 10.23** (Right) *Pityriasis versicolor presenting as hypopigmented patches after exposure to sunlight. The normal skin tans, but not that affected by fungus.*

responsible for causing persistent pruritus ani, and if this is appreciated and the condition correctly treated, the very distressing symptom may be cured.

### Treatment

Until recently oral erythromycin was the most effective treatment, as the organism was highly sensitive. However, topical sodium fusidate ointment is also effective.

## Moniliasis

*Candida albicans* is a yeast-like parasite which differs from a true yeast in that it forms a pseudo-mycelium and does not reproduce by budding. *C. albicans* most commonly affects the skin and mucous membranes but it can also cause systemic disease, such as gastroenteritis, endocarditis, septicaemia and meningitis. It is important, however, to remember that it exists most commonly on the skin and mucous membranes and in the gastrointestinal tract without giving rise to pathological change at these sites. In addition isolation of the organism from a diseased skin may not mean that candida is the cause of the disorder, but may be merely coincidental. Candida, however, will seed itself in pre-existing pathological conditions and under these circumstances is a secondary invader and may give rise to further pathological change. The exact circumstances under which it becomes virulent and gives rise to disease are not known but often there is an underlying condition whether it be local or systemic.

Cases of moniliasis as seen by the dermatologist may be divided into those affecting the skin and those affecting the mucous membranes or muco-cutaneous regions.

Like ringworm fungi, moniliasis is frequently found in moist areas of the skin. In most instances, however, there is usually a predisposing cause for the infection.

### Intertrigo

Monilial intertrigo is usually found in the submammary, perianal and perivulval skin. It presents as erythematous macerated skin in these areas and can be distinguished from simple seborrhoeic eczema because there are satellite lesions (Figures 10.24 and 10.25). The skin involvement may spread onto the buttocks or down the thighs (Figure 10.25). In monilial intertrigo at these sites, particularly in females, it is most important to test the urine for sugar as monilial vulvitis is one of the common presenting features of diabetes mellitus.

A fairly common site for infection of the skin with monilia is the space between two fingers (Figure 10.26) but not usually the feet as with ringworm. The condition presents as erythema, peeling and maceration of the skin on the sides of the two adjacent fingers. It can be distinguished from eczema of the hands since the lesion is frequently solitary and unilateral.

### Treatment

Ideally the diagnosis should be established by demonstrating the organism either by microscopy or culture. If there is any underlying cause for the skin involvement, such as diabetes, it must be treated otherwise local treatment will not be successful. There is no systemic therapy for cutaneous moniliasis but topical preparations are effective. Nystatin is

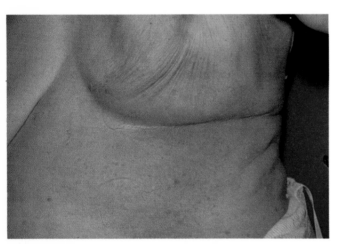

**Figure 10.24** *Monilial intertrigo in the submammary region. Satellite papules extend on to the trunk beyond the intertriginous area.*

**Figure 10.25** *Monilial intertrigo in the groins and on the vulva. Satellite papules are visible extending on to the medial side of the thigh.*

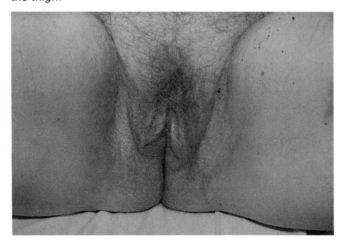

**Figure 10.26** *Monilial infection between two fingers.*

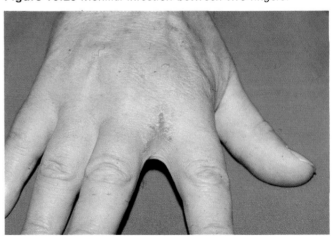

a highly effective preparation against candida albicans (it has no action against ringworm fungi). The newer preparations, clotrimazole and miconazole nitrate, are also effective against candida albicans as well as ringworm fungi. One of the advantages of using nystatin is that it is available combined with a topical steroid in proprietary preparations. It is helpful to combine the anti-monilial drug with corticosteroids as there is usually inflammatory change in the skin. As in other types of intertrigo, the areas affected should be kept as dry as possible. Daily painting with Pig. Magenta is often helpful, and this substance also has weak anti-monilial properties. However, painting with magenta is not always cosmetically acceptable to the patients.

### Monilial Paronychia

This disorder is sometimes referred to as 'barmaids' disease'. It occurs predominantly in people who have their hands in and out of water during the course of the day, and it is therefore, much commoner in women than men. The underlying cause is thought to be damage and a break in the cuticle due to a 'chapping' effect. The organisms then gain entry into the posterior nail fold.

The paronychia may be subacute at first with pain, swelling and redness of the posterior nail fold (Figure 10.27) from which a small quantity of pus may be seen exuding. Later, the paronychia tends to become chronic with swelling and some slight redness of the posterior nail fold and loss of the cuticle (Figure 10.28), but the condition is not painful. If it persists, as it usually does, there is secondary dystrophy of the nail plate because the nail matrix is affected (Figure 10.28). The nail dystrophy usually appears first at the lateral margins of the nail plate with a brownish green discolora-

tion (Figures 10.28 and 10.29). Subsequently, the whole of the plate may be involved. In the first instance only one or two fingers will be affected but others will become involved if preventive measures are not taken.

### Treatment

The most important measure is to keep the hands as dry as possible to prevent growth of the organism and allow healing of the nail fold to occur. Patients must be instructed to wear rubber gloves with cotton gloves inside for all household duties and for their work if it involves having their hands in water. Topical measures are helpful but not curative if the fingers are continuously immersed in water. Nystatin cream should be applied to the nail fold twice daily but patients should be instructed not to 'push' the ointment under the nail fold otherwise further damage to the reforming cuticle will occur. Painting with anti-fungal lotions is sometimes helpful, and may be preferable to using creams. The older lotions, e.g. gentian violet and magenta paint, would not be cosmetically acceptable on the fingers, but there are available many colourless proprietary preparations. The paint should be applied after the hands have been washed. Occasionally bacteria are also present in chronic paronychia of the fingers and if the organism can be isolated a short course of the appropriate antibiotic applied topically or even given systemically may be helpful. Removal of the nail is not indicated and should be avoided.

### Oral Mucocutaneous Moniliasis

Moniliasis of the mouth is often referred to as thrush. The characteristic appearance is creamy white patches on the

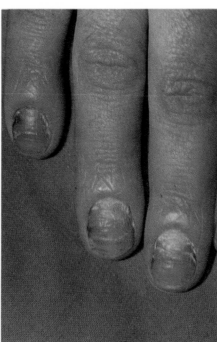

**Figure 10.28** *Chronic monilial paronychia. There is swelling of the posterior nail fold, loss of the cuticle, deformity of the nail plate, and greenish-brown discoloration at the sides of the nail.*

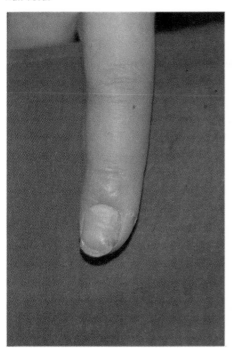

**Figure 10.27** *Monilial paronychia. There is redness and swelling of the posterior nail fold.*

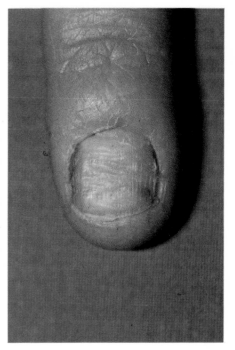

**Figure 10.29** *Monilial paronychia. There is ridging of the nail and characteristic greenish-brown discoloration at the sides of the nail plate.*

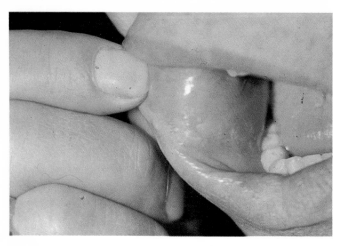

**Figure 10.30** *Candida albicans infection on the buccal mucosa of the mouth appears as yellowish-white patches.*

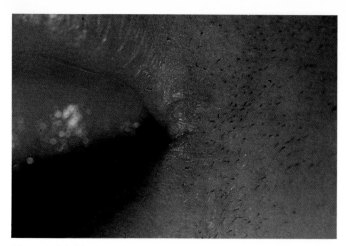

**Figure 10.31** *Angular stomatitis presents as 'cracks' at the corners of the mouth. Secondary infection with monilia may occur.*

mucous membranes of the mouth (Figure 10.30). The white patches are easily removed to reveal a red base. There may be only a few scattered patches on the tongue, cheeks, palate or gums, but in more severe instances they may extend to involve the oesophagus and upper respiratory tract. Occasionally candida infection is seen at the angles of the mouth, angular stomatitis (perlèche). However, not all cases of angular stomatitis are due to candida (Figure 10.31). The presence of candida is easily confirmed by examination of the material from the white patches.

Thrush is most commonly seen in young infants. However, it does appear to be a complication of broad spectrum oral antibiotics, the theory being that the alteration which occurs in the bacterial flora of the alimentary canal after administration of these antibiotics allows overgrowth with candida. This may be too simple an explanation and host immunity is probably also an important point in the development of pathological lesions. Recently, underlying abnormal immune mechanisms and disorders of calcium and iron metabolism have been reported in persistent cases of oral cutaneous candidiasis.

### Treatment

Nystatin is the treatment for oral moniliasis. In children a suspension of nystatin can be administered as drops. Nystatin tablets are available and in older patients should be held in the mouth in the hope of achieving a high enough concentration to produce a cure. In angular stoma-titis due to monilia, nystatin cream should be used. If cases are proving resistant to treatment then the patients should be investigated to exclude deficiencies in their immune mechanisms or underlying abnormalities of calcium and iron metabolism.

### Monilial Vulvo vaginitis

The same general principles which apply to oral thrush hold equally well for vaginal candidiasis. The organism is often present in the normal vagina, more frequently during pregnancy, while taking the contraceptive pill, or after antibiotic therapy. There is an increased incidence of monilia in women with pathological conditions of the cervix and vagina.

Moniliasis of the vagina is characterised by a white or yellow 'curdy' discharge. This is associated with pruritus vulvae. The vulval area becomes red and swollen and a white discharge is present. The condition may subsequently spread to give rise to a macerated eczema of the perineum, peri-vulval skin and groins (Figure 10.25).

### Treatment

Initial treatment with nystatin vaginal pessaries at night should be commenced. If the skin is also affected this should be treated as described above for monilial intertrigo. The urine should be tested for sugar, and a search made for any predisposing gynaecological condition.

# 11. Viral Infections

### Warts

W ARTS represent a very common viral infection of the skin. The wart virus affects the epidermal cell, causing cellular proliferation and excess keratin production. Thus the viral wart is a small tumour on the skin with a thickened rough surface (Figure 11.1). The appearance of the wart, however, varies depending on the site involved.

Histologically warts are composed of finger-like processes of epidermis with dermal capillaries extending up between these processes. These capillaries come very close to the surface and are often a useful diagnostic point. If the surface of the wart is pared with a scalpel bleeding points may be seen (Figure 11.2). On other occasions the vessels are thrombosed and are seen as small black dots in the wart (Figures 11.2 and 11.3). This appearance has sometimes led to the mistaken diagnosis of a malignant melanoma.

Warts, being a viral disease, are contagious. However they are not as contagious as is commonly supposed and infection of several members of a family is not common. Immunity to the wart virus is probably important in determining whether the virus causes clinical lesions.

Before deciding on the treatment of warts the natural history of the condition must be appreciated. The vast majority of warts will undergo spontaneous resolution in the course of time. However this period varies from a few months to a few years and as yet there is no way of predicting how long warts may last if left untreated. Since there is no drug effective against the wart virus, treatment is empirical. Warts are epidermal structures and therefore if they undergo spontaneous remission they will leave no scar or mark. Thus too radical treatment, which involves damaging the dermis, should be avoided at all costs. Treatment may be divided into radical and palliative.

### Radical Treatment

All the radical procedures described below are aimed at removing or destroying the actual tumour. None of the procedures has a 100 per cent success rate, even in the best hands. The results will depend on a number of factors, the two most important being: a) that the procedure is carried out properly and b) the degree of host immunity that the patient has to the wart virus at the time the procedure is carried out.

**Figure 11.1** *Typical warts. Raised lesions with a rough hyperkeratotic surface and clefts.*

**Figure 11.2** *Wart after paring. The bleeding point seen is an enlarged capillary and the black dots thrombosed capillaries.*

**Figure 11.3** *Wart with characteristic black dots, which are thrombosed capillaries.*

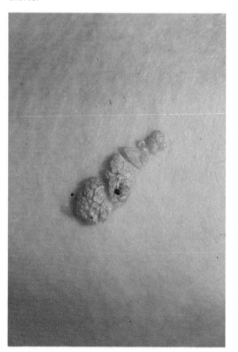

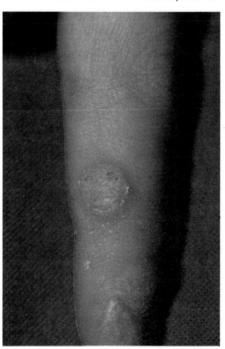

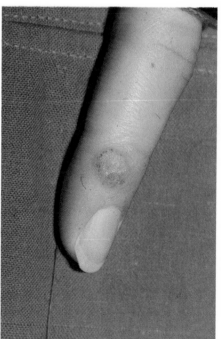

*a) Curettage and cautery:* This should be done under local anaesthetic. The wart is scooped out with a small curette and the base and edges of the ulcer produced by curettage are cauterised, to stop the bleeding and to destroy any cells which contain wart virus which may have been left after curettage.

*b) Carbon dioxide snow or liquid nitrogen:* These substances work on the principle that when applied to the skin for the appropriate length of time they will produce a subepidermal blister and the epidermis (which contains the wart) will be shed. The length of time for which they are applied to the skin will depend on the site involved and size of the lesion treated.

*c) Podophyllin:* This is a cytotoxic agent which will destroy epidermal cells (and therefore the wart virus) by topical application. The strength of the podophyllin used and the medium in which it is used will depend on the site of the lesion.

*d) Formalin:* This is only suitable for treatment of plantar warts.

*e) Escharotics:* The most commonly employed are nitric acid and trichloracetic acid. However the results are not predictable and there may be severe burning of the surrounding tissues.

*f) Surgery and radiotherapy:* These are mentioned only because they are to be found in the older text books on the treatment of warts. Neither is justifiable for the treatment of such a benign and self-limiting disorder.

### Palliative Treatment

If, as often occurs, warts are numerous, none of the above measures is really suitable. Painting with salicylic acid, which is a keratolytic, in a suitable base will tend to break up the excess keratin on the surface of the lesion and make the wart less conspicuous. Simple occlusion with airtight plasters for six to eight weeks (the plasters are changed weekly) tends to cause maceration of the epidermis, and this may lead to the destruction of the wart.

In some instances placebo therapy is required and there are reports of its success. However, whether it is a true placebo effect or simply the natural history of the lesion which causes the disappearance of the wart is not really known.

### Warts on the Hands

This is one of the commonest sites for warts. They may occur on the palms or dorsa of the hands, and they may be numerous (Figure 11.4) or solitary. The lesion usually presents as a small hyperkeratotic papule, usually 2–5 mms. in diameter (Figure 11.3). However, occasionally they may be larger. If the warts occur on the skin around the nails they may simply present as thickening and rough skin on the nail

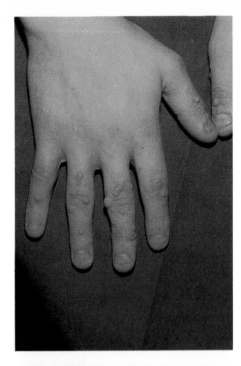
**Figure 11.4**
*Numerous warts on the hands.*

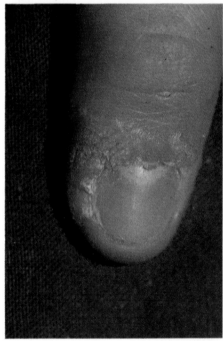
**Figure 11.5**
*Periungual warts – roughened, thick skin on the nail folds.*

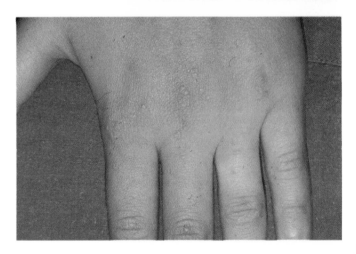

**Figure 11.6** (Right) *'Flat warts' on the back of the hand.*

folds (Figure 11.5). On the back of the hands they may appear as small, brown, just palpable, lesions (sometimes referred to as plane or flat warts) (Figure 11.6).

### Treatment

Treatment for warts on the hands is usually sought for cosmetic reasons or because the lesion is at a site which interferes with the patient's work. In the first instance simple painting with 10 per cent salicylic acid in collodion should be tried. If the lesion is not showing any signs of spontaneous cure after two to three months and the patient is still asking for further treatment, then this should be decided on the number of lesions present. If the wart is solitary or there is only a small number then treatment with carbon dioxide snow, liquid nitrogen, or curettage and cautery will probably give the best result. If the warts are numerous the patient will have to continue with palliative or placebo measures. If the warts are periungual, curretage and cautery is best avoided, particularly if the warts are on the posterior nail fold, for permanent damage to the nail bed may follow. Periungual warts often respond to podophyllin applied under occlusive strapping. The podophyllin at this site is best used in an ointment base. The ointment is applied weekly and the plasters changed only weekly. If the podophyllin cannot be tolerated then simple occlusive strapping should be tried for six to eight weeks. Cryotherapy with liquid nitrogen or carbon dioxide snow is suitable for periungual warts although the treatment may have to be carried out more than once. The interval between treatments should be two to three weeks.

### Plantar Warts

The sole of the foot is another very common site for warts. These are often referred to as verrucae by the patients. The commonest presentation of plantar warts to the doctor is usually as a result of a school inspection of the feet. The other reason for presenting is because the wart is on a weight bearing part of the sole of the foot and causes pain.

Warts on the soles of the feet do not present as small raised papules, because the pressure on the sole forces the lesion into the dermis and thus causes pressure on the nerve endings, giving rise to pain. The typical plantar wart is a flat, circular hyperkeratotic lesion (Figure 11.7). There is often gross hyperkeratosis over the surface of the lesion, making it difficult to distinguish it from a simple callosity. In these instances the lesion should be pared with a scalpel. If it is a callosity only uniform thickened keratin will be found, if it is a wart capillary bleeding points or the clefts between the finger-like processes of the structure will be seen.

Warts on the soles of the feet may be solitary or multiple. Occasionally there may be a group of warts which involves a confluent area on the sole of the foot. These are sometimes referred to as 'mosaic warts' (Figure 11.8).

### Treatment

The simplest treatment, and effective if carried out correctly, is formalin soaks. Five per cent formalin solution should be poured into a saucer or flat dish and the part of the sole where the wart or warts are situated soaked in this lotion for

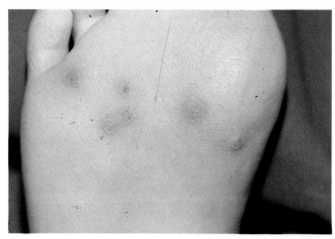

**Figure 11.7** *Plantar warts. They are not usually raised above the skin surface because of pressure on the sole of the foot.*

**Figure 11.8**
*Mosaic wart on the sole. The area of involvement is large and confluent.*

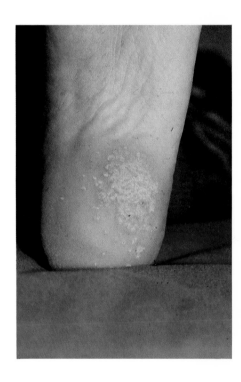

**Figure 11.9** *Typical warts on the chin.*

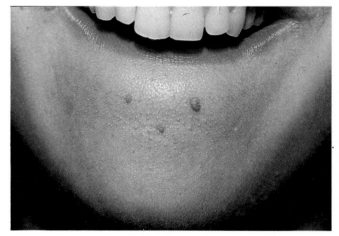

15 minutes daily. If the wart is near the toes and the formalin is likely to go between or under the toes then these places should be protected by applying vaseline before soaking in formalin. If this is not done then the skin may become fissured and sore at these sites. The treatment should be continued for at least a month and the hyperkeratotic dry skin pared away before each soak to allow the lotion to penetrate to the deeper parts of the wart. If after a month's treatment, properly carried out, there is no improvement, the strength of the formalin should be increased to 7 per cent and subsequently, if necessary, to 10 per cent. It is usually easy to see if the treatment is being carried out regularly because the skin in contact with the formalin becomes dry and flaky.

If formalin therapy is not successful and the lesions solitary or few, then curettage and cautery or cryotherapy may be used. If the lesions are on the toes they should be treated as described above for periungual warts on the fingers. Mosaic warts appear to be particularly resistant to treatment, possibly because of the extent of the lesions. This implies little or no immunity to the wart virus, and thus the lesions persist.

### Warts on the Face and Trunk

The face and neck are the next commonest sites for warts, after the hands and soles of the feet. Warts on the face may either present as the typical, rough, scaly papule (Figure 11.9) or they may appear as flat, plane warts (Figure 11.10) similar to those on the back of the hands. In children warts are frequently seen on the lips, due to sucking fingers which have warts on them. On the lips the warts present as smooth white papules. On the neck and in the beard area warts are usually seen as grouped papules probably due to auto-inoculation during shaving (Figure 11.11).

#### *Treatment*

Strong acids, podophyllin, and formalin should not be used for the treatment of warts on the face. If the lesions are unsightly or causing difficulty with shaving in a man, then the treatment of choice is cauterisation. In the case of numerous flat warts palliative treatment with a solution containing 3 per cent salicylic acid should be used. Other agents which cause the skin to peel, such as sulphur or resorcinol, may also be used.

### Peri-anal and Genital Warts

In these moist areas the spread and growth of the warts may be very rapid, so it is extremely rare to find solitary or only a few lesions (Figure 11.12). The warts are raised above the skin.

#### *Treatment*

The most effective and simplest treatment is to paint the lesions with a 25 per cent solution of podophyllin in either spirit or tinct. benz. co. The surrounding skin should be protected with vaseline. The patient should be instructed to wash off the podophyllin after six to eight hours. The treatment should be carried out weekly. In the majority of cases the warts will disappear after a few 'paintings' but in others

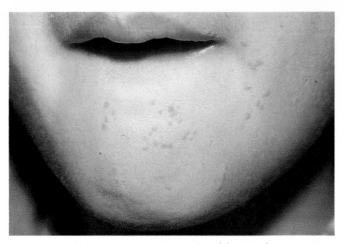

**Figure 11.10** *Flat, plane warts on the chin, another presentation of warts on the face. The lesions often have a light brown colour.*

**Figure 11.11** *Numerous warts in the beard area. The warts may be spread by shaving.*

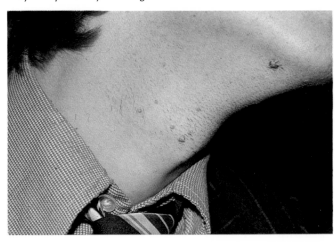

**Figure 11.12**
*Warts on the vulva and peri-anal skin. Warts tend to be numerous in these moist areas.*

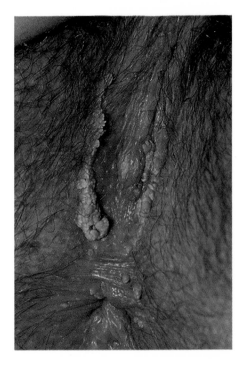

66

the lesions may prove resistant to treatment, although their size and number is controlled. Reinfection of the skin is common if the warts are also present in the anal canal or vulva and vagina. In these instances it may be necessary to ask for the assistance of the appropriate surgeon to cauterise the lesions. Care must be taken not to cause scarring.

## Molluscum Contagiosum

Molluscum contagiosum is another viral tumour of the skin. It is most commonly seen in children but does occur in adults. Auto-inoculation is common and the lesions are usually multiple and grouped on a particular part of the body (Figure 11.13). The individual lesion has a characteristic appearance; it is a small, bulbous, sessile papule, the surface of which is umbilicated (Figure 11.14). The lesion is 'pearl' coloured (Figure 11.15), but when there is secondary bacterial infection it is red due to inflammation.

Although auto-inoculation is common, it is rare to find more than one member of the household with the complaint at any given time.

### Treatment

The lesions, as far as is known, do not undergo spontaneous clearance. However, anything which interferes with the architecture of the individual lesion induces resolution. Thus slight trauma or secondary infection will often result in cure. Treatment is relatively easy. One of the simplest methods is to pierce the lesion with a sharpened pointed orange stick which has been dipped in 1 per cent phenol. No local anaesthetic is required for this procedure, and it is relatively painless. The lesions should clear without leaving a scar as a molluscum is entirely due to epidermal proliferation.

### Orf

This is a virus infection of the skin which is caught from contact with sheep. The lesions, which are nearly always on the hands, consist of inflammatory papules which subsequently become haemorrhagic and pustular; they are usually less than 1 cm in diameter, although there may be a surrounding area of erythema. The differential diagnosis is primary (accidental) vaccination, anthrax, and erysipeloid. The lesions undergo spontaneous resolution within a few weeks; there is no specific treatment.

### Milker's Nodules

This is similar in appearance to orf, but the infection is acquired from cows. The initial lesions usually occur on the fingers and may be multiple or single. They attain their

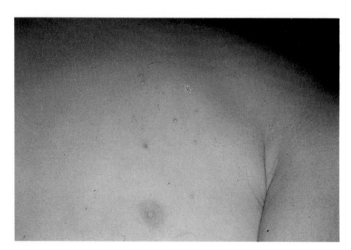

**Figure 11.13** *Grouped lesions of molluscum contagiosum.*

**Figure 11.14** *Molluscum contagiosum lesion showing central umbilication.*

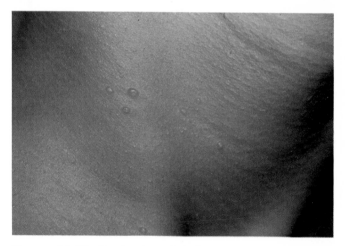

**Figure 11.15** *Pearl-coloured lesions of molluscum contagiosum.*

**Figure 11.16** *Herpes simplex. A group of small blisters on an erythematous base.*

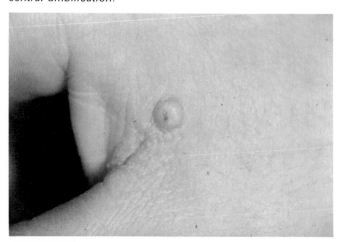

maximum size within two weeks in the form of brownish firm nodules which are usually 1 cm in diameter, but may be larger. The lesions are painless and not pustular. No treatment is required unless there is bacterial infection.

## Herpes Simplex

The characteristic clinical lesion produced by the herpes simplex virus on the skin is a group of blisters on an erythematous base (Figure 11.16). The commonest site for herpes simplex is on the lips or around the mouth, but the skin lesions may appear anywhere. Very rarely the virus may affect the internal organs and cause systemic illness, or a generalised skin eruption in patients with atopic eczema.

The time of the initial infection with the herpes simplex is rarely determinable (unless the primary illness is severe) but almost all of the population eventually becomes infected as evidenced by the regular presence of neutralising antibodies to the herpes simplex virus.

The commonest site affected is the lips (herpes labialis). The appearance of the blisters is often preceded by a tingling and burning sensation, as it is thought that the virus lives in the nerve endings of the skin, and these are affected by the virus as it becomes active and migrates into the skin. Herpes simplex infection of the lips may be precipitated by an illness with a high fever (herpes febrilis) or after exposure to the sun or wind. The first visible lesion is a group of small blisters (Figures 11.17 and 11.18). These may become pustular (Figure 11.19) after two to three days and then rupture to form a crust (Figure 11.20) and finally a scab (Figure 11.21). Complete healing of the lesion usually takes from ten to fourteen days after the appearance of the blisters. The lesions of herpes simplex may occur repeatedly, with the shortest interval between attacks being as little as six weeks. The lesions usually appear at the same site in recurrent herpes simplex, and this has been attributed to the virus remaining in the skin or nerves innervating this particular area. However the virus has never been demonstrated in the skin between the episodes of clinical involvement but it can be shown to be present in the blisters.

One of the commonest reasons for misdiagnosing herpes simplex at sites other than the lips is failure to realise that the virus may produce lesions at other sites. Although the face (apart from the lips) is frequently involved, the eruption may appear anywhere on the skin (Figures 11.22 and 11.23).

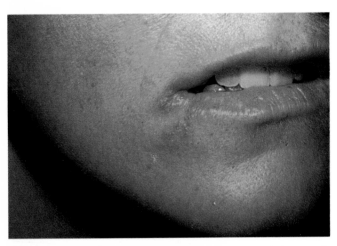

**Figure 11.17** *Group of small blisters at the side of the mouth at an early stage of herpes simplex infection.*

**Figure 11.18** *Blisters on the upper and lower lip in extensive herpes simplex infection.*

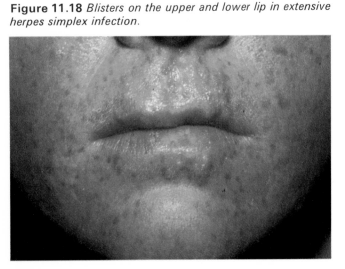

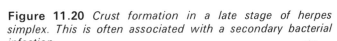

**Figure 11.19** *Pustules forming in the intermediate stage of herpes simplex infection.*

**Figure 11.20** *Crust formation in a late stage of herpes simplex. This is often associated with a secondary bacterial infection.*

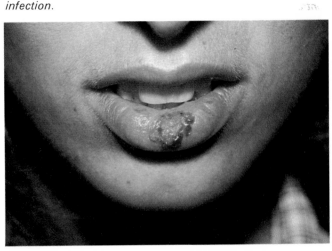

68

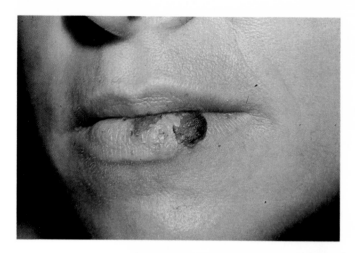

The clinical presentation is that of grouped blisters, often in a discoid pattern. The blisters often have an erythematous base, may become pustular (Figure 11.23), and subsequently form a crust before healing. The next commonest site, after the lips, to be affected by herpes simplex is the genitalia, particularly in males. The virus which causes the genital lesions can be differentiated from that affecting the skin elsewhere. The virus causing the genital lesions is known as herpes virus II and that causing lesions elsewhere herpes virus I. The clinical sequence of events in genital herpes simplex is the same as that elsewhere. There is the prodromal symptom of a tingling or burning sensation, then blisters (Figure 11.24) followed by pustules and finally erosions (Figure 11.25) rather than scabs. Herpes simplex of the genitalia is often recurrent and the diagnosis can be established by taking swabs from the lesions in the blistering stage for virological examination.

Herpes simplex very occasionally affects the fingers and is often misdiagnosed as a bacterial infection, as the condition is painful and may give rise to redness and swelling before the blisters are apparent (Figure 11.26). Herpes simplex affecting the fingers is termed 'the herpetic whitlow' and is common in nurses who have been caring for patients with a tracheostomy; the virus is thought to inhabit the respiratory tract without causing lesions.

### Complications

The commonest complication is secondary bacterial infection. Repeated herpes simplex infection at one particular site may cause scarring, especially if there is superadded bacterial infection. Herpes simplex infection in the periocular region may spread on to the eye where it may give rise to corneal ulcers.

*Primary gingivostomatitis and vulvovaginitis.* This type of clinical response to primary infection is rare. Why it occurs in some and not others is not understood. At the onset of the infection there are no antibodies to the virus, but these appear in high titre as the disease progresses. When the mouth is involved, as occurs most frequently in young children, painful oral lesions develop, associated with fever, malaise and lymphadenopathy. White patches appear in the mouth with surrounding erythema. Ulcers may eventually form. Redness and swelling of the gingiva are characteristic of the infection. In the female, vulvovaginitis may occur with white plaques on the vaginal wall and cervix. Subsequently these areas may ulcerate. In both gingivostomatitis and vulvovaginitis the characteristic blisters may occur on the surrounding skin.

*Eczema herpeticum (Kaposi's varicelliform eruption).* This is a widespread vesicular eruption, with lesions predominantly on the face (Figure 11.27), occurring in persons who have atopic eczema. Clinically, the disorder is indistinguish-

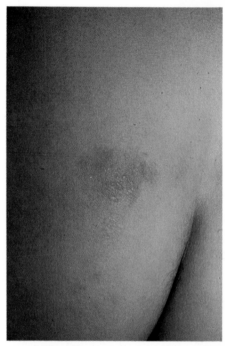

**Figure 11.22**
*Herpes simplex infection on the back of the upper arm.*

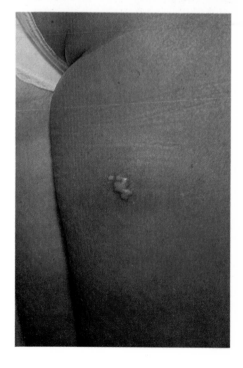

**Figure 11.23**
*Pustule formation in herpes simplex infection on the back of the thigh.*

able from eczema vaccinatum (the eruption which occurs in atopic subjects after vaccination against smallpox).

*Systemic herpes simplex infection* may occur. The commonest and most serious site of involvement is the central nervous system.

## Diagnosis

This can usually be made on clinical grounds alone. In the more difficult cases virological studies can be helpful in establishing a diagnosis. The virus can be found in the blister fluid and can be cultured. Rising antibody titre can be demonstrated during the infection.

## Treatment

In the majority of instances no treatment is required.

Patients often ask for something and astringent lotions, e.g. spirit, can be given for topical use in the blistering stages of the eruption. If secondary bacterial infection occurs then topical antibiotics should be given. The organism most likely to cause secondary infection is the staphylococcus and sodium fusidate ointment is likely to be the most effective.

Recurrent herpes simplex infection is a considerable problem for the patient, particularly if the attacks are frequent. The anti-viral drug idoxuridine is effective against the herpes simplex virus. However, because of the nature of skin lesion it is difficult for the drug to penetrate the skin in order to kill the virus and stop progression of the lesion. The drug is too toxic for parenteral use for routine purposes. The drug has to be used in the initial stages, i.e. when the prodromal symptoms of burning or tingling occur. To allow idoxuridine to penetrate the epidermis it must be made up in a special solvent. The standard solvent used is dimethyl sulphoxide. Initially 5 per cent idoxuridine in dimethyl sulphoxide is used. The lotion should be applied by a brush to the affected area every two hours for the first two days. Once the blisters rupture there is no point in continuing the applications. Although idoxuridine in dimethyl sulphoxide is not a cure for recurrent herpes simplex, it does seem to lessen the severity of the attacks. Unfortunately painting the affected area between attacks to try to eradicate the virus has not been successful.

### Herpes Zoster (Shingles)

Skin lesions due to herpes zoster virus occur in the area of skin supplied by one particular sensory root ganglion. Prior to the appearance of the skin lesions there may be severe pain for two to three days in the area supplied by the parti-

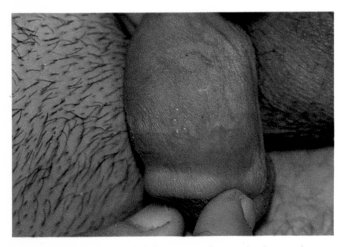

**Figure 11.24** *Grouped blisters on the penis due to herpes simplex.*

**Figure 11.25** *Erosion on the penis in an advanced herpes simplex infection.*

**Figure 11.26** *Herpetic whitlow.*

**Figure 11.27** *Eczema herpeticum. Widespread herpes simplex infection in a subject with atopic eczema.*

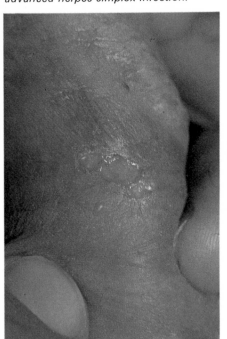

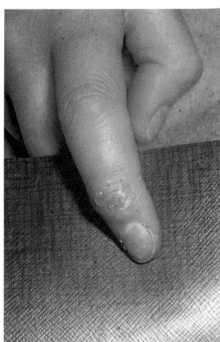

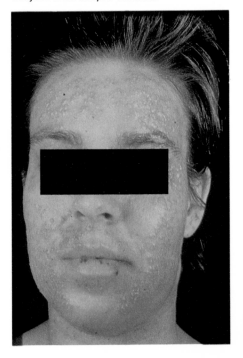

cular nerve root, and this may in some cases give rise to diagnostic problems.

The skin lesions are small blisters with some surrounding erythema (Figure 11.28). They may occur in one or two small groups (Figure 11.29) or they may occur throughout the area of skin innervated by the particular sensory root ganglion involved (Figures 11.30, 11.31 and 11.32). New groups of lesions may appear over a period of a few days after the first lesions have appeared. The blisters tend to be larger (up to 1.0 cm diameter) than in herpes simplex and not infrequently are haemorrhagic (Figures 11.31 and 11.32).

Herpes zoster most commonly affects the thoracic nerves. The appearance is characteristic with lesions extending from the spine on the back (Figure 11.29) to the midline on the anterior chest (Figure 11.30) or abdominal wall in the front (Figure 11.31). The lesions do not usually cross the mid-line.

Herpes zoster may affect the root ganglia of the sensory nerves. The fifth cranial nerve is the most commonly affected and usually only one division, i.e. ophthalmic, maxillary or mandibular, is involved (Figure 11.33). If the ophthalmic division is affected (Figure 11.34), keratitis and conjunctivitis may occur in addition to the skin lesions. In the otic type of zoster, in which the geniculate ganglion is involved, there may be an accompanying Bell's palsy and skin lesions in the external auditory canal, on the pinna and on the tongue.

### Complications

Generalised herpes zoster may occur as a very widespread eruption. In these instances there is usually a severe underlying disturbance of the patient's immune mechanisms such as in a reticulosis. Generalised herpes zoster is sometimes the presenting manifestation of Hodgkin's disease or leukaemia and patients must be investigated for these conditions.

Chicken-pox and herpes zoster are caused by the same virus and in some patients the two diseases may occur together. Secondary infection of the blisters does occur but is not as common as in herpes simplex lesions, perhaps because herpes simplex more commonly affects the lips.

Post-herpetic neuralgia is one of the most distressing symptoms that occurs after the skin lesions have subsided. The complication is seen more frequently in elderly patients, and may last for years. Paralysis of the skeletal muscles, not

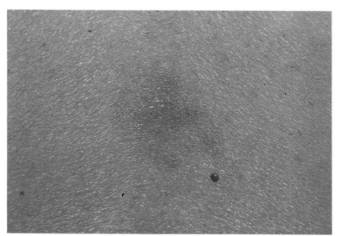

**Figure 11.28** *Early lesions of herpes zoster. Small blisters and papules on an erythematous base (similar to herpes simplex).*

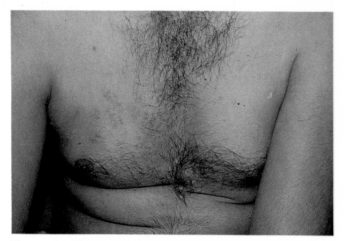

**Figure 11.30** *Lesion of herpes zoster showing involvement of the skin supplied by an intercostal nerve. The lesions do not as a rule cross the mid-line of the body.*

**Figure 11.31** *Grouped haemorrhagic blisters affecting the dermatome supplied by a posterior root ganglion. The lesions are unilateral.*

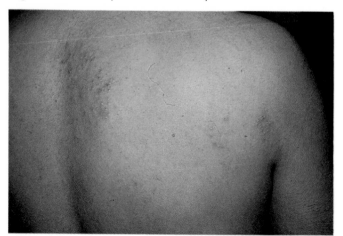

**Figure 11.29** *Grouped lesions of herpes zoster.*

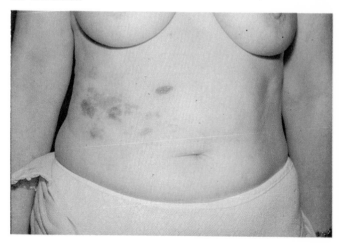

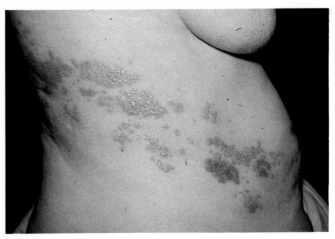

**Figure 11.32** *Haemorrhagic blisters in herpes zoster, with localisation of the eruption to a dermatome supplied by one posterior root ganglion.*

**Figure 11.33** *Herpes zoster infection of the skin supplied by the mandibular division of the fifth cranial nerve.*

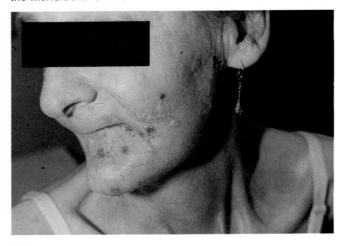

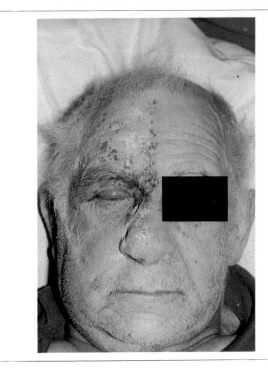

**Figure 11.34** *Herpes zoster. Involvement of the ophthalmic division of the fifth cranial nerve.*

usually permanent, can occur due to the herpes zoster virus. The muscles involved are usually those supplied by the same nerve root as that in which the sensory root is involved.

### Diagnosis

The disease is usually easy to diagnose on clinical grounds once the blisters have appeared. However, if there is difficulty the virus can be isolated and grown from the blister fluid and identified by virological tests.

### Treatment

In the majority of patients only palliative treatment is required e.g. mild analgesics. If secondary infection of the blisters occurs then topical antibiotics are required. Pain during and after the active stage of the disease may be very severe and stronger analgesics may be needed. Drugs of addiction, e.g. pethidine and the opiates, should be avoided because of the possible lengthy duration of post-herpetic neuralgia.

Systemic corticosteroids and Vitamin $B_{12}$ injections have been advocated in herpes zoster in an attempt to shorten the course of the disorder and prevent post-herpetic neuralgia. However neither of these preparations have been shown conclusively to prevent post-herpetic neuralgia.

Corticosteroids may be helpful in reducing the inflammatory response, particularly if the eye is involved. The management of ophthalmic herpes zoster, however, should be supervised by an ophthalmologist. Five per cent idoxuridine in dimethyl sulphoxide used in the blistering stage (the same regime as for herpes simplex) has been advocated by some. It has been reported to shorten the duration of the disorder and lessen the severity and incidence of post-herpetic neuralgia. However, these claims are not proven and this treatment should probably be reserved for special circumstances. It must be stressed that the cost of using idoxuridine in dimethyl sulphoxide for herpes zoster (particularly if the lesions are extensive) would be considerable.

# 12. Bacterial Infections

ALTHOUGH bacterial infections of the skin still result in an appreciable number of attendances in a dermatological clinic, their incidence has fallen over the last two decades because of the advent of antibiotics and general improvement in hygiene and the standard of living.

## Impetigo

This is one of the commonest bacterial infections seen today, and is unfortunately often misdiagnosed before attending the skin clinic.

Impetigo is usually caused by *Staphylococcus aureus* but it is not uncommon to find a mixed infection with a staphylococcus and a β-haemolytic streptococcus. It is important to understand that streptococcal infections of the skin may give rise to renal and cardiac complications, in the same manner that streptococcal infections of the upper respiratory tract may give rise to pathological manifestations which are not respiratory in nature.

### Morphological Appearances

Impetigo is an infection of the epidermis. In the early stages

a purulent blister (Figures 12.1 and 12.2) may be the first sign of the disorder. However, because the roof of the blister is so thin, it very soon ruptures and impetigo frequently presents as superficial erosions (Figures 12.3, 12.4 and 12.5). Another form of presentation is the golden crusted lesion which is caused by seropurulent weeping which clots and combines with keratin to form crusts (Figures 12.6 and 12.7). Satellite lesions are common in impetigo and appear around the older and larger lesions (Figures 12.1, 12.4 and 12.8). Original lesions may also coalesce to form large eroded or crusted areas. The hands and face are the commonest sites for impetigo and this is probably because of the easy spread from one to the other. The diagnosis of impetigo should be considered when there is asymmetry of the lesions (Figure 12.8), unlike the endogenous eczemas. Frequently the diagnosis may be made more difficult because of the prior use of topical steroids, which alter the classical appearance of the lesions by diminishing the crusts and the golden appearance of the lesions.

### Treatment and Management

Impetigo is a contagious disorder and, thus, care over per-

**Figure 12.1** *Impetigo. Small, superficial pustules, the initial lesion surrounding the more typical crusted lesion.*

**Figure 12.2** *Blisters in impetigo. The edges of the blister are visible, and the centre of the lesion is beginning to ulcerate.*

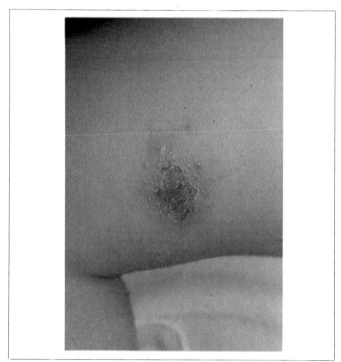

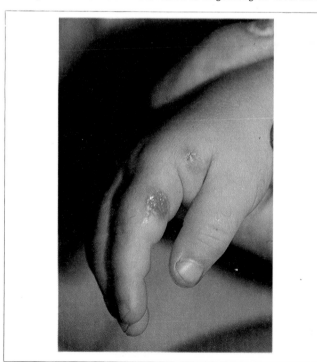

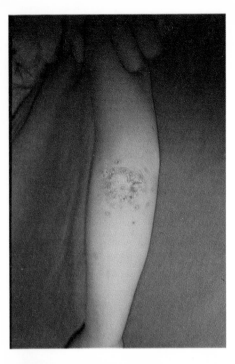

**Figure 12.3**
*Superficial erosions and blister formation in impetigo.*

**Figure 12.4**
(Below)
*Erosion with edges of blister and small satellite lesions in impetigo.*

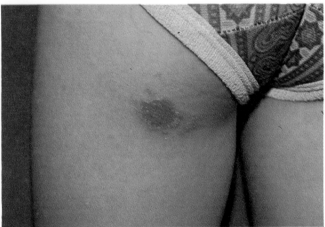

**Figure 12.5**
*Erythematous erosions and superficial crusts in impetigo.*

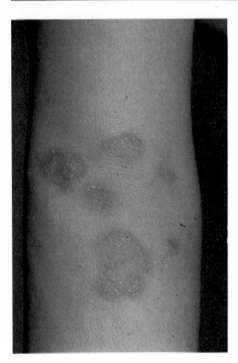

sonal hygiene is important. Children should be kept away from school until cured.

It is important that the 'crusts' are removed by soap and water before the application of topical antibiotics, as otherwise the antibiotics will fail to penetrate in a high enough concentration to the depth where the bacteria are to be found. Impetigo is an epidermal disorder and topical antibiotics are usually all that is required. Systemic antibiotics are rarely required in impetigo, but if the condition is very extensive a course of penicillin should be given. The choice of topical antibiotic varies with physicians. The most commonly used topical antibiotics are fusidic acid and neomycin. These are both highly effective against most strains of staphylococcus aureus and B-haemolytic streptococcus. Neomycin is often combined with bacitracin in proprietary preparations. The ointment should be applied at least three times a day and continued until all signs of the disorder have cleared.

In patients in whom the impetigo recurs, or when it involves the nostrils, it is highly likely the organism is harboured in the anterior nares and the topical antibiotic should also be applied to this site.

### Ecthyma

This is essentially a deep type of impetigo. It usually begins as a small pustule which erodes through the epidermis and into the upper dermis to produce a shallow ulcer. Oozing occurs with formation of a firm yellow crust.

The commonest site is the legs and lesions may occur repeatedly after minor trauma. Because of the involvement of the dermis, healing leaves a superficial scar. Poor hygiene and neglect are predisposing factors.

### Treatment

As there is involvement of the dermis, systemic as well as topical antibiotics should be used. The choice of antibiotics is empirical until the results of bacteriological investigations are available.

### Secondary Impetigo

This is where primary skin disease is secondarily infected with staphylococci and streptococci and clinical lesions, as seen in primary impetigo, are formed. The commonest skin disease to become secondarily infected is eczema. The treatment is as for impetigo, in the first instance, and the eczema is treated subsequently. In secondary impetigo the infection may involve the dermis because of existing skin disease and in these instances systemic antibiotics are also required if the condition is to be quickly controlled.

### Folliculitis

Bacterial infection is only one of the causes of a folliculitis. Folliculitis on the back is often seen in association with or as a manifestation of seborrhoeic eczema.

Folliculitis today is most commonly seen in the beard area in persons who shave (Figure 12.9). It is commoner in Negroes than Caucasians and is thought to be caused by short curling hairs which grow back 'into' the skin and set up irritation with secondary infection. Persons who use cutting

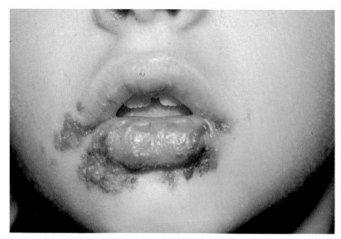

**Figure 12.6** *Thick, yellow crusts in impetigo. Some exudation is seen.*

**Figure 12.7** *Dry, yellow crusts in impetigo.*

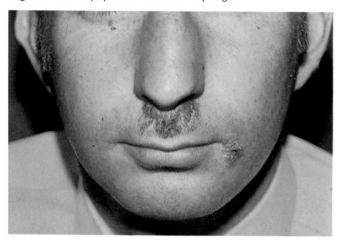

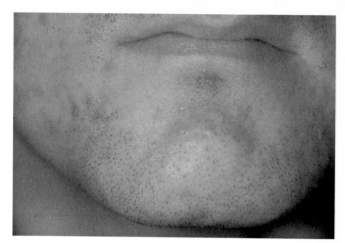

**Figure 12.9** *Folliculitis of the beard area.*

oils are liable to develop a folliculitis if the area is continually soaked with the oil (Figure 12.10).

### Treatment

If the folliculitis is associated with seborrhoeic eczema, treatment as for eczema is often all that is necessary to cure the disorder. In some instances further improvement is obtained with weak keratolytic preparations such as 2 per cent salicylic acid in spirit or a cream base. Folliculitis of the beard area is often difficult to clear other than by not shaving. If the patients do not wish to grow a beard topical antibiotics should be used on the area after swabs have been taken to determine the sensitivity of the organisms. The antibiotic should be applied to the anterior nares in addition to the beard area.

### Furuncles (Boils)

This is essentially a folliculitis but the infection spreads well away from the follicle into the surrounding dermis. Clinically, the lesion begins as a small, red nodule which increases in size and becomes fluctuant within two to three days. During this time the lesion becomes 'walled off' in the dermis. The apex of the lesion ultimately becomes yellow (pus) and breaks down and discharges pus and necrotic tissue. When the lesion heals a small scar is left. A 'carbuncle' is a coalescent aggregation of a number of furuncles and ultimately gives rise to a deep, pus-filled ulcer. Pathologically, the abscesses around the hair follicles are not walled off from each other.

The commonest site for furuncles and carbuncles is the back of the neck, although they may occur at any site which has hair follicles.

### Treatment

For a single, isolated boil no treatment, other than 'hot compresses', is required. If the lesion is fluctuant, pain can be relieved by a small incision through the centre of the lesion. Topical antibiotics are of no therapeutic value in the treatment of the lesion.

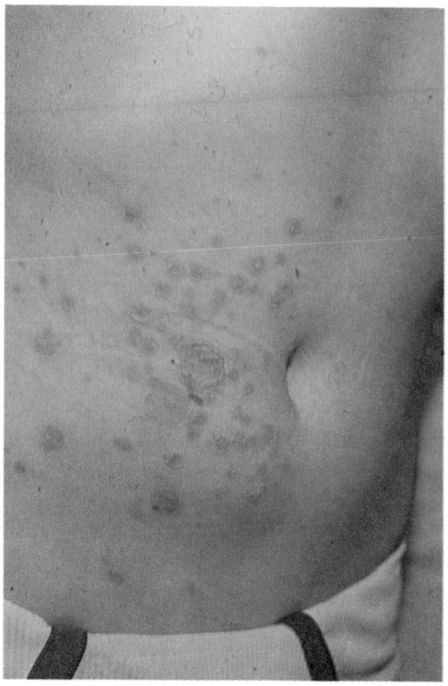

**Figure 12.8** *Asymmetry of the eruption in impetigo.*

## Multiple and Recurrent Boils

The commonest cause for recurrent boils is the harbouring of the infecting organism in the anterior nares, axillae or perineum. Swabs should be taken from these sites. The appropriate topical antibiotics should be applied twice daily for at least a month to the area where the organism has been found. Bathing with 30 ml of 10 per cent hexachlorophane added to the bath water has been claimed to be of some value in decreasing the number of lesions when multiple boils are present. Systemic antibiotics are helpful in the early phase of the lesions and will prevent new lesions forming. However, unless the underlying source of the organisms is found, systemic antibiotics will not prevent the development of new lesions when the antibiotics are stopped. In all cases of recurrent skin infections it is wise to think of underlying systemic disease. The commonest systemic diseases to present with skin infections are diabetes mellitus and reticuloses. Rarer disorders, such as the dysgammaglobulinaemias, should be considered as a last resort.

### Erysipelas

This is a streptococcal infection which has become relatively uncommon. It begins as a red, indurated plaque of cellulitis with a distinct border. As in other forms of cellulitis the skin feels hot. There is usually constitutional upset and fever. The commonest sites to be affected are the face and scalp, the portal of entry being a small crack in the skin of the nostril or external auditory canal. However, if the patient has had any previous wounds or other dermatoses (Figure 12.11), these are obvious portals of entry for the organism. Occasionally, erysipelas is recurrent at one particular site, e.g. on the face, and may eventually leave brawny permanent oedema. The cause for this recurrent infection may be a chronic otitis externa.

#### Treatment

Systemic antibiotics, usually penicillin, are required. The affected part, particularly if it is a limb, should be rested. If the disorder is recurrent it is worth looking to see if there is a persistent portal of entry in the form of a chronic dermatosis which requires treatment.

### Tuberculous Skin Infections

As with tuberculosis at other sites of the body, infections of the skin have become increasingly rare. A number of clinical varieties of skin tuberculosis have been described in the past and these clinical descriptive terms will be adhered to.

#### Lupus Vulgaris

This was probably the commonest form of skin tuberculosis seen in the past. The lesion may occur at any site on the skin, although it is most frequently seen on the hands and neck. It presents as a reddish-brown nodular plaque (Figure 12.12) and, when pressed with a glass spatula, small

**Figure 12.10**
*Oil folliculitis on the forearm.*

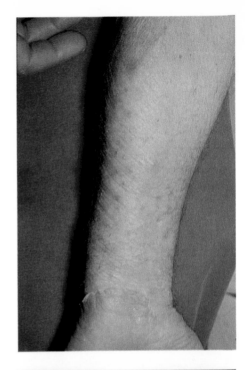

**Figure 12.11**
*Erysipelas. Deep infection caused by a streptococcus which gained entry via eczema on the hand. The erythematous lesion has a sharply demarcated edge.*

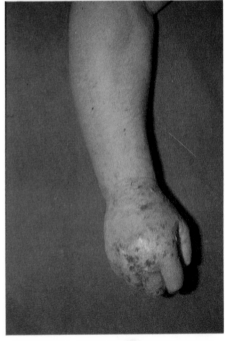

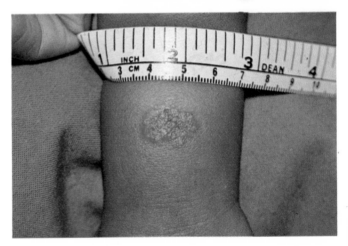

**Figure 12.12** (Right) *Lupus vulgaris. Reddish nodular plaque on the forearm.*

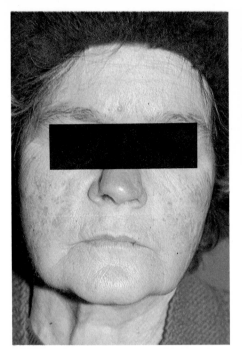

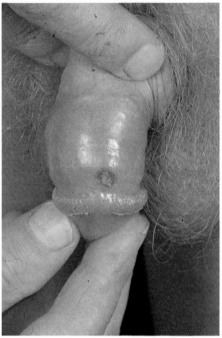

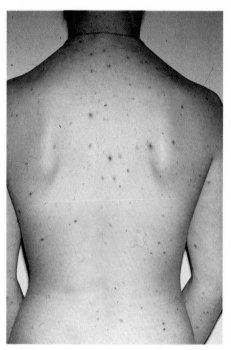

**Figure 12.13** *Scarring on the cheeks following lupus vulgaris.*

**Figure 12.14** *Primary chancre on the penis.*

**Figure 12.15** *Scattered papular eruption in secondary syphilis.*

brownish nodules (so-called apple-jelly nodules) can be seen. The surface of the lesion may be scaly but usually the lesion presents as an infiltrated plaque, as the primary changes are in the dermis. If untreated, the disease is progressive and leads to destruction of the tissues and subsequent scarring (Figure 12.13). In the past it has led to severe disfigurement.

### Tuberculosis Verrucosa Cutis

This is another clinical form of tuberculosis. It results from direct inoculation of the skin with tubercle bacilli. It may be granulomatous with superficial pustules and may well be misdiagnosed as a 'chronic boil'. Another appearance is that of granuloma with a 'warty' surface.

### Scrofuloderma

This is an extension of tuberculous infection to the skin from an underlying focus in bones or lymph nodes.

### *Treatment*

The therapy for tuberculous infections of the skin is the same as that for tuberculous infections at other sites of the body. However, in lupus vulgaris the chronicity of the condition and its non-contagious nature make streptomycin unnecessary and PAS and isoniazid are all that is required.

### Syphilis: Primary Lesion or Chancre

The typical lesion is a painless ulcer with an indurated border usually less than 1 cm in diameter (Figure 12.14). There is accompanying regional lymphadenopathy. The commonest sites for a chancre are naturally on the penis and vulva. However, for a high proportion of women it is present on the cervix and, therefore, may well escape de-

**Figure 12.16**
*Extensive papular eruption in secondary syphilis.*

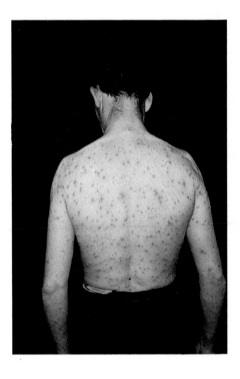

tection. The chancre may appear anywhere on the skin, the most frequent extragenital sites being the lips, mouth, fingers, breasts and anus.

### Secondary Syphilis

Lesions of secondary syphilis may appear within six weeks and up to one year after initial infection. The commonest form of skin lesion is a reddish papular eruption on the trunk and limbs (Figures 12.15, 12.16 and 12.17). The

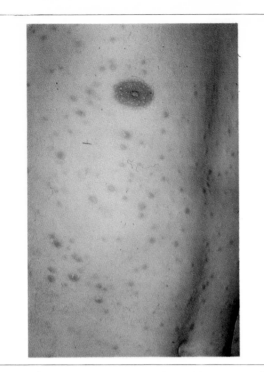

Figure 12.17 *Reddish-brown papules with some scaling in secondary syphilis. This eruption is similar to guttate psoriasis.*

Figure 12.19 *Secondary syphilis. Condylomata lata on the peri-anal skin.*

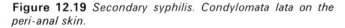

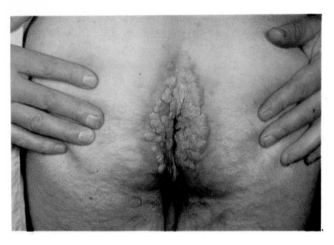

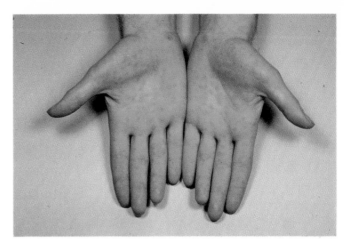

Figure 12.18 *Papular eruption on the palms in secondary syphilis. This is a helpful clue to the diagnosis as this type of eruption does not occur in eczema, psoriasis or pityriasis rosea.*

Figure 12.20 *Secondary syphilis. Condylomata lata on the vulva and perineum.*

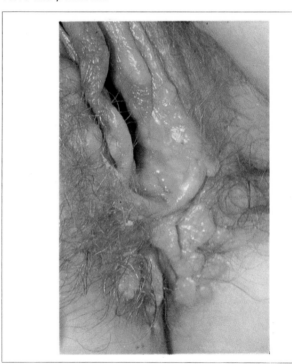

lesions may be very widespread (Figure 12.16) or few in number (Figure 12.15). A not infrequent site to be involved is the palms of the hands and involvement at this site can sometimes be helpful in the clinical diagnosis (Figure 12.18). At first the lesions may be discrete papules but on occasions they will merge giving a confluent scaly dermatosis similar to psoriasis or eczema of the palms. On the genitalia or around the anus, small eroded exudative papules (condylomata lata) (Figures 12.19 and 12.20) may be seen and may have to be distinguished from viral warts—particularly if they are the only manifestation of secondary syphilis. Secondary syphilitic eruption of the skin was always considered to be the great mimicker of other dermatoses. Most

frequently it resembles psoriasis or pityriasis rosea, but in any atypical dermatosis of recent onset secondary syphilis should be remembered (Figure 12.21).

Hair loss may occur in secondary syphilis. This is usually patchy and the areas affected are not completely bald, as occurs in alopecia areata.

The mucous membranes may also be involved in secondary syphilis. In the mouth and pharynx there are oval, round (Figure 12.22) or arcuate greyish patches which tend to ulcerate and may give rise to the classical 'snail-track' ulcer.

Accompanying the cutaneous lesions of secondary syphilis there may be constitutional upset and lymph-

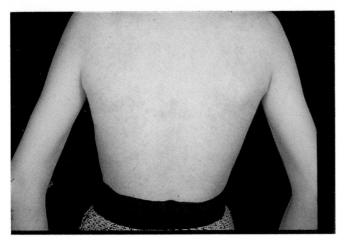

**Figure 12.21** *Non-specific, generalised, erythematous eruption in secondary syphilis.*

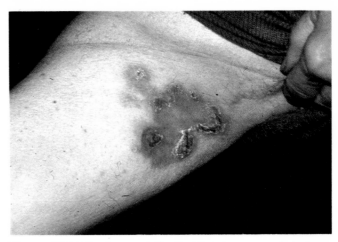

**Figure 12.23** *Tertiary syphilis. Reddish-brown, scaly lesion.*

**Figure 12.22** *Round, greyish-white patches on the oral mucosa in secondary syphilis.*

**Figure 12.24** *Tertiary syphilis. Glossitis with secondary leukoplakia.*

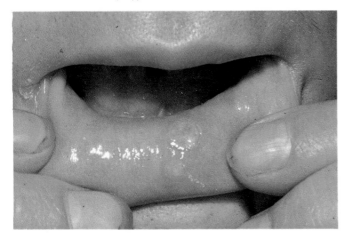

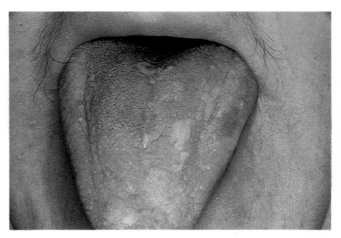

adenopathy. Serological tests are always positive in the secondary stage of syphilis.

### Tertiary Syphilis

Only the skin manifestations of tertiary syphilis will be mentioned. All are very rare today. Nodular lesions of varying size (2 mm–5 mm) of a reddish brown colour usually appear in groups and spread out in varying directions to produce lesions of irregular pattern (Figure 12.23).

### Gumma

This is a mass of syphilitic granulation tissue. It begins below the skin but extends into the skin. The lesions are painless and slow-growing but frequently break down and ulcerate.

### Chronic Interstitial Glossitis

This appears as extensive and irregular fissuring of the tongue with accompanying leukoplakic changes (Figure 12.24).

### *Treatment*

Penicillin is still the drug of choice for the treatment of syphilis. It is best for patients with primary and secondary syphilis to be treated in venereology departments so that 'contacts' can be traced and patients investigated for the possibility of other venereal diseases.

# 13. Drug Eruptions

IN this chapter the skin lesions produced by drugs taken or given systemically will be considered, as opposed to skin lesions produced by topically applied therapeutic agents. Almost any drug can produce a skin eruption, and this may mimic most dermatological entities, or produce bizarre patterns of reaction in the skin. In dealing with a patient who presents with a rash it is most important to find out, as part of the history-taking, whether the patient has received in the immediate past, or is receiving at the present time, any drugs. It also is very important to appreciate that what the patient means by 'a drug' and what the doctor means are often very different, and specific questions may have to be asked. The patient usually considers 'drugs' only as those substances prescribed by a doctor for a serious or acute illness. But it must be remembered that many drugs such as mild analgesics (salicylates and phenacetin), laxatives and 'tonics' can be bought by patients over the pharmacy counter without any prescription from a doctor. These substances may also cause drug eruptions but are not considered to be drugs by the patient. In addition, any drug which may have been taken for any length of time, e.g. regular hypnotics, tranquillisers, or contraceptive pills are not considered 'drugs' by the patient or thought likely to have been responsible for his complaint, because he has been taking the drug for a long time without any previous trouble. Thus in practice it is better to ask the patient whether he takes any pills, tablets or medicines of any description for any complaint, rather than saying 'Have you taken any drugs recently?'. Both patient and doctor must appreciate that even if the drug has been taken for any length of time without causing previous trouble it should not be immune from suspicion of causing the present complaint.

Despite the wide variation in pattern of reaction that may be produced in the skin, there are some guide lines to suggest that a drug may be the cause.

1. The eruption is frequently widespread because it is produced by a circulating agent as opposed to a topically applied substance.

2. It commonly appears as an inflammatory response with widespread pruritus.

3. It is usually of sudden onset.

4. It may be associated with constitutional upset such as

**Figure 13.1** *Angioneurotic oedema around the eyes due to penicillin.*

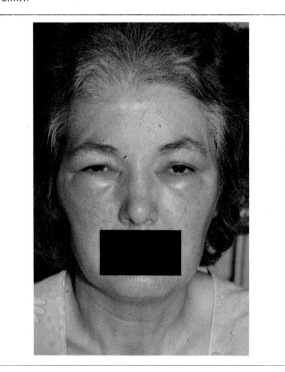

**Figure 13.2** *Urticaria due to penicillin sensitivity.*

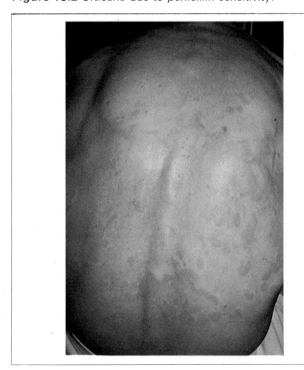

malaise or fever, and there may be signs of disorder of other organs frequently affected by drugs such as the bone marrow, liver, or kidneys.

It is not possible to be definitive about which drugs cause a specific pattern of skin reaction but certain drugs are more likely than others to cause recognised dermatological entities and the following significant examples of eruptions should be considered as possibly due to drugs if a positive history is obtained.

### Types of Drug Eruptions

*Urticaria and angioneurotic oedema.* The two commonest drugs to cause angioneurotic oedema (Figure 13.1) and urticaria (Figure 13.2) are penicillins and salicylates. The urticaria due to penicillin usually appears one to two weeks after starting the drug, but may occur as long as six weeks after commencement. Urticaria following penicillin may be persistent and last for many weeks. Other drugs which may cause urticaria are thiouracil, isoniazid, vaccines, serum and quinine.

*Exanthem or morbilliform eruption.* This is a widespread macular erythematous eruption (Figure 13.3). Latterly there may be some scaling or peeling (Figure 13.4) or occasionally the lesions are raised with an urticarial appearance. At the present time the commonest cause of this type of eruption is ampicillin. Other drugs which also cause this pattern are phenylbutazone, gold, para-amino salicylic acid (PAS), phenothiazines and barbiturates.

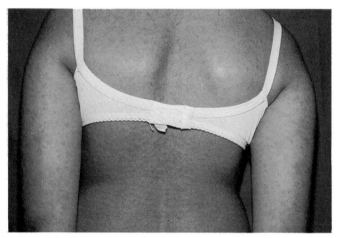

**Figure 13.3** *Widespread erythematous, macular, and a few urticarial, lesions due to ampicillin sensitivity.*

**Figure 13.4** *End stage of ampicillin skin rash, with reddish-brown scaling in a symmetrical pattern.*

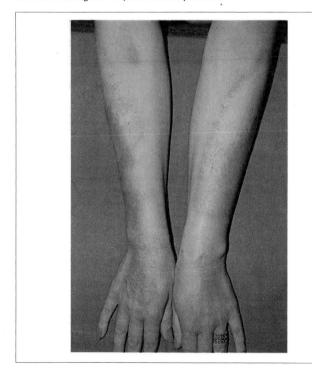

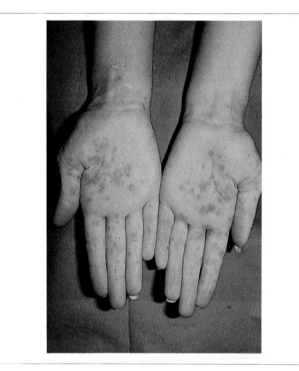

**Figure 13.5** *Erythema multiforme on the hands caused by sulphonamides.*

**Figure 13.6** *Ulceration of the lips and oral mucosa in erythema multiforme.*

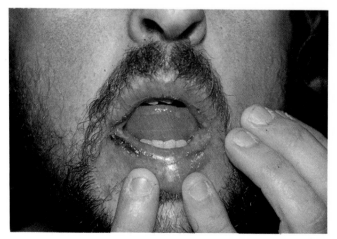

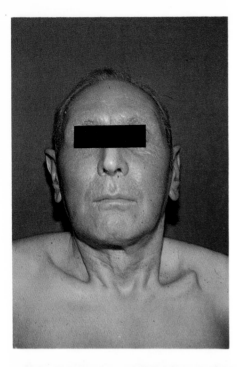

**Figure 13.7**
*Acute photosensitivity eruption due to dimethyl chlortetracycline.*

**Figure 13.8**
(Below) *Photosensitivity due to chlorpromazine.*

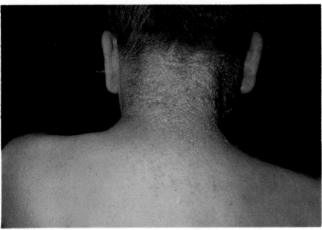

**Figure 13.9**
*Bullous drug eruption after sulphonamide administration.*

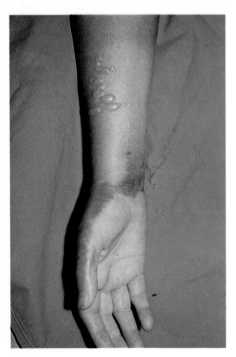

*Erythema multiforme.* This is a well-recognised dermatological entity with annular erythematous and vesicular lesions occurring predominantly on the extensor surfaces of the hands (Figure 13.5), forearms and feet. There may also be oral lesions (Figure 13.6) usually presenting as ulcers or erosions on the mucous membrane. This type of eruption is most commonly caused by sulphonamides and penicillin.

*Photosensitivity.* This is usually an acute erythematous eruption on light-exposed areas (Figures 13.7 and 13.8) and in some instances the inflammation may be so intense as to produce blistering of the skin. The drugs most likely to be responsible are the phenothiazines, particularly chlorpromazine, and the tetracyclines. It is also well recognised as a reaction to the sulphonamides, quinidine, and the chlorothiazides.

*Blistering eruptions.* The commonest drugs to produce large discrete blisters in the skin (Figure 13.9) are the sulphonamides, but they have also been described after penicillin, barbiturates and phenylbutazone.

*Purpura.* Purpura (Figure 13.10) is most commonly seen on the legs whatever the basic cause, and drug-induced purpura is no exception. It may occur following phenylbutazone, quinidine, chloramphenicol, sulphonamides and barbiturates.

*Erythema nodosum.* This presents as painful reddish indurated plaques, usually on the front of the legs (Figure 13.11). It can be drug induced, and the sulphonamides seem to be the commonest drugs to cause this type of eruption.

*Generalised or exfoliative dermatitis.* This is essentially an eczematous response of the skin (Figure 13.12). Heavy metals are the commonest cause and gold is probably the only 'heavy metal' which is still used in clinical practice. This eruption has also been noted after phenylbutazone, barbiturates, quinine and sulphonamides.

*Lichen planus-like eruptions.* These are sometimes very similar to lichen planus but are usually more confluent (Figure 13.13) and slightly scaly. The eruption in these instances is referred to as lichenoid. The drugs which have been implicated are gold, chloroquine, mepacrine, para-amino salicylic acid and amiphenazole.

*Acne.* This is a well recognised complication of systemic corticosteroid therapy. It is also induced by iodides, bromides, tridione and some of the current oral contraceptives. In the latter instance the acne appears to be due to the relative dominant effect of the progesterone component of the contraceptive on the sebaceous glands.

*Lupus erythematosus.* A lupus erythematosus-like syndrome has been induced by drugs. Apart from the classical cutaneous lesions (Figure 13.14), internal organs are also involved and LE cells and positive anti-nuclear factor are found. The first drug found to cause this reaction was the

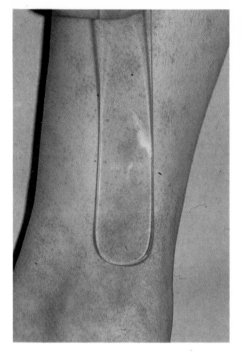

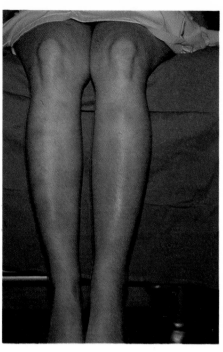

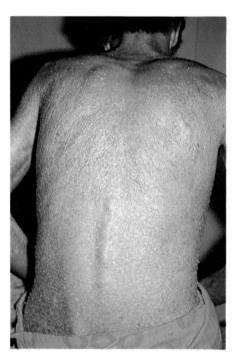

**Figure 13.10** *Purpuric eruption on the leg after phenylbutazone therapy.*

**Figure 13.11** *Erythema nodosum caused by sulphonamides.*

**Figure 13.12** *Exfoliative dermatitis following gold therapy.*

hypotensive agent, hydrallazine. Procaine amide and penicillin are now also known to precipitate lupus erythematosus.

*Pigmentation.* Of the modern drugs, oral contraceptives are the most likely to produce pigmentation. This is very similar to the chloasma type of pigmentation seen in pregnancy (Figure 13.15), and may be due to the same mechanism. The pigmentation is distributed on cheeks and forehead.

*Pruritus ani and pruritus vulvae.* This is seen as a complication of broad spectrum antibiotics. Monilia is often present in the skin in these instances, and it is thought to be due to altered bacterial flora.

*Fixed drug eruptions.* These follow highly distinctive clinical patterns. They consist of circumscribed lesions which reappear at exactly the same site each time the drug is taken. The clinical lesions are variable but usually consist of an erythematous patch with possible urticarial or bullous formation and an erosion may follow (Figure 13.16). This usually subsides within a few days, but residual pigmentation may persist for a considerable length of time. Fixed drug eruptions by their very nature usually occur only with drugs which are taken infrequently for if the patient was on continuous medication the eruption would be present continuously in the active stages. The drugs most frequently concerned are barbiturates and phenolphthalein which is found in a number of proprietary laxative preparations.

It is usually accepted that any drug can cause an eruption as a possible side effect and from what has been said it would appear that any drug may produce nearly any type of skin reaction.

### Mechanism of Drug Eruptions

*Allergy.* It is usually assumed by doctor and patient alike that if a patient develops a rash after taking a drug then he is 'allergic' to it. However, the varied pattern of drug eruptions and their subsequent behaviour and the fact that antibodies cannot be detected to these drugs suggests that not all drug reactions are allergic in nature.

*Toxic.* It would appear from the behaviour of many of these reactions that they exert a direct damaging effect on the skin, but the exact biochemical processes involved are not known.

*Idiosyncrasy.* This is a term used when a patient develops a severe reaction even when a small dose of the drug is given. This may be due to abnormal enzyme systems in the body, which do not exist in the majority of individuals.

*Intolerance.* Most drugs are either metabolised by the tissues, usually liver, or excreted unchanged by the kidney. Thus, if these organs have impaired function and the particular drug is not excreted or metabolised by them, it may accumulate in the body to toxic levels and cause a reaction, which it would not have done in a healthy individual. If it is known that a patient has liver or kidney disease care must be taken before prescribing any drug until it is known that there is no risk from the drug or its breakdown products.

### Diagnosis

The diagnosis of drug reactions may prove difficult. Often the only way of making the diagnosis is on circumstantial evidence. The clinical picture is still the most useful guide; the time relationship between taking the drug and the

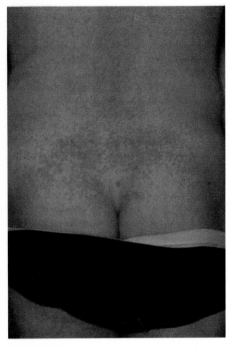

**Figure 13.13** *Lichenoid eruption due to para-amino salicylic acid.*

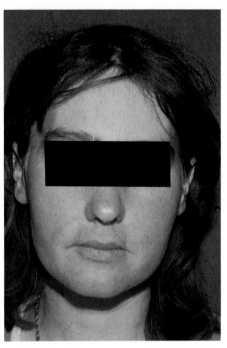

**Figure 13.14** *Systemic lupus erythematosus syndrome after penicillin therapy.*

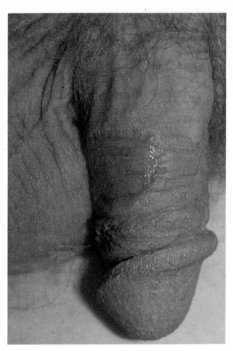

**Figure 13.16** *Fixed drug eruption. Erosion on penis after initial blister formation, due to a sulphonamide. The lesion occurs at the same site each time the drug is taken.*

**Figure 13.15** *Pigmentation on cheeks, forehead and upper lip due to oral contraceptive.*

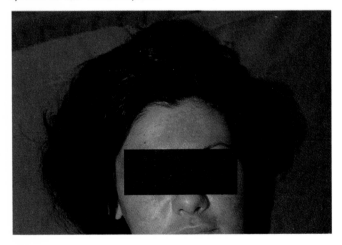

development of the rash is very important, as is the pattern of reaction produced. Unfortunately, there are no safe or reliable tests for substantiating a diagnosis. Intradermal or patch tests are useful only if there is a 'true allergy' and even then there is a high incidence of false negatives. In addition if a patient has an allergy to a drug such as a penicillin then even a small dose given intradermally may prove fatal. An oral test dose of the drug is sometimes suggested after the rash has cleared, but this carries the possibility of inducing an even more severe reaction. Laboratory in vitro tests with the patient's serum and drug have been tried but the number of false negative results is so high at present that the tests are of very little practical value.

## Management and Treatment

Once a drug is suspected of causing an eruption it should be stopped. The treatment is dependent on the type of eruption but is largely symptomatic. If there is severe pruritus then systemic antihistamines should be given in adequate dosage. If there is an inflammatory response in the epidermis with erythema and scaling, topical steroids may be helpful. Systemic steroids may also be valuable in appropriate cases.

In certain instances when it is considered necessary to use the drug again, desensitisation has been tried. The drug is given to begin with in very small quantities so that no reaction is produced and the dose is then gradually increased. The procedure does not always work and is not without risk.

The question will always be raised, did the drug actually cause this eruption and must it always be avoided in the future? If there is a *definite* history of a reaction following a particular drug and other drugs can be used as alternatives then it is probably advisable to avoid the 'incriminated' drug unless it is a question of life and death. There have been slight anomalies in the past when a drug which appeared definitely to have caused an eruption induced no reaction when given again. In some instances it is now known that the disease process for which the drug is being given can combine with the drug to produce the reaction. Yet when the drug is given on a second occasion for a different disease no reaction occurs. This has been recorded with ampicillin, e.g. when it is given in glandular fever.

# 14. Bullous Disorders

ALTHOUGH many disease processes affecting the skin (e.g. bacterial infections, viral infections, vasculitis) may cause blisters, there is a group of rare diseases in which the predominant sign is blisters. These diseases are usually known as the 'bullous disorders'. These are pemphigus, pemphigoid, dermatitis herpetiformis, epidermolysis bullosa and herpes gestationis. Although all the conditions are rare they are well recognised dermatological entities and no comprehensive discussion of dermatological conditions would be complete without mention of them.

## Pemphigus

The word pemphigus comes from the Greek pemphix meaning pustule. Pemphigus occurs in middle aged and elderly patients, appearing more commonly in members of the Jewish race. It is most important to appreciate that pemphigus affects not only the skin but also the mucous membrane of the mouth, pharynx and vagina, and one third of patients with pemphigus may present with lesions at these sites before developing lesions on the skin. Pemphigus has no specific predilection for site of involvement and may present anywhere on the skin. The lesions tend to become widespread in a short space of time.

Pemphigus is an epidermal disease, and the disorder is one of failure of the epidermal cells (keratinocytes) to adhere together and maintain cell contact. The cells drift apart and the space between the cells fills with fluid which eventually gives rise to a blister. Because the blister forms *in* the epidermis the roof of the blister is very thin and ruptures easily. There are a number of clinical presentations of pemphigus depending on whether the disease process is occurring high up or low down in the epidermis. When blisters are present in pemphigus they tend to be flaccid because of their thin roof which ruptures easily giving rise to erosions (Figure 14.1). Crusting of the eroded surface of the skin soon occurs, and thus patients may present with one of three types of skin lesion—blisters, erosions or crusted, scabbed lesions, or a combination of any two of these (Figures 14.2, 14.3 and 14.4). Occasionally pemphigus presents with widespread erosions only (Figure 14.5), and this form of the disease may be misdiagnosed unless it is appreciated that pemphigus may present without blisters. When pemphigus affects the mucous membranes of the mouth, the pharynx or the genital tract in females, it presents as red, denuded areas or superficial ulcers (Figures 14.6 and 14.7), and no blisters are seen. In patients who have persistent erosions in the mouth, pemphigus has to be considered in the differential diagnosis.

## Aetiology

Pemphigus is now considered to be one of the so-called auto-immune diseases. The antibody which is found in pemphigus is formed against the 'intercellular substance' of the epidermal cells. Thus the epidermal cells do not

**Figure 14.2** *Pemphigus. Three types of lesion are present, blisters, erosions and crusted scabs.*

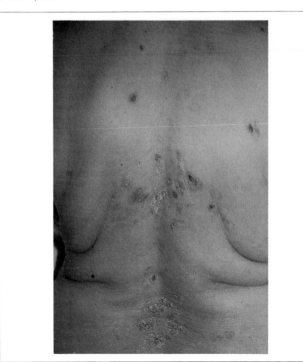

**Figure 14.1** *Blisters and erosions in pemphigus.*

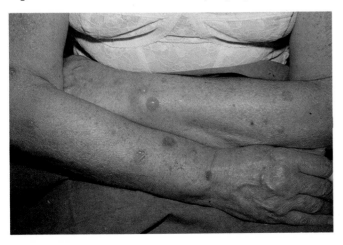

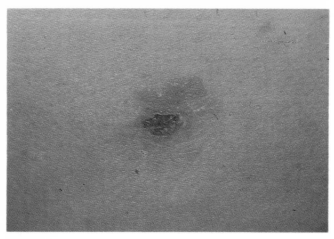

**Figure 14.3** *Thin roofed blister and an adjacent crusted lesion.*

**Figure 14.4** *Erosions and crusted, scabbed lesions in pemphigus. No blisters are present.*

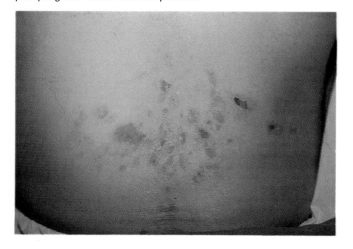

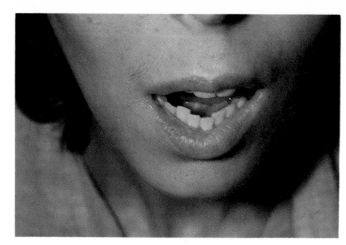

**Figure 14.6** *Persistent erosions on the mucosal surface of the lips in pemphigus.*

**Figure 14.7** *Erosions on the hard palate in pemphigus.*

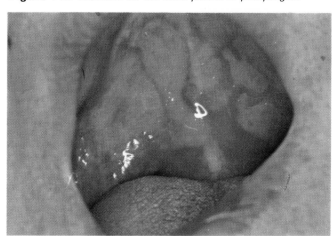

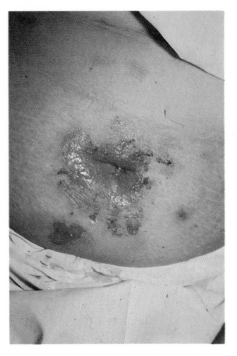

**Figure 14.5**
*Pemphigus presenting as acute, weeping, superficial erosions. Again no blisters are present.*

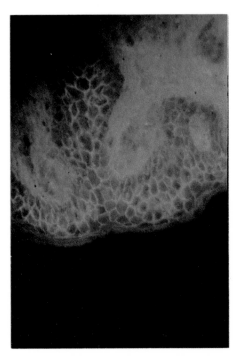

**Figure 14.8**
*Localisation of antibody to the 'intercellular substance' in pemphigus. The bright green pattern in the epidermis reveals the presence of antibody.*

adhere to each other and drift apart, with blister formation and destruction of the epidermis. The detection of the antibody is now one of the diagnostic tests in pemphigus. The antibody is found in the skin adjacent to the lesions and also circulating in the blood. The antibody can therefore be detected by direct (in the skin) or indirect (in the serum) studies. Usually a fluorescent technique is used (Figure 14.8). Although, as in all auto-immune disorders, it is not known whether the antibody is primary or secondary, remissions and relapses in pemphigus can be forecast by the amount of antibody in the serum, and this is helpful in the management of the patient.

### Treatment

Prior to the advent of corticosteroids, pemphigus was invariably a fatal disease. In pemphigus topical treatment is not effective and the steroids have to be taken orally. Unfortunately large doses of steroids are required, and thus it is imperative that the diagnosis is confirmed, by histological and immunological tests, before treatment is started. The initial dose of steroid is usually in the order of 100 mg prednisone daily until the disease is brought under control and no new lesions are appearing. The dose is then gradually reduced to a maintenance level which will stop further outbreaks of the disorder. The maintenance dose of prednisone varies from patient to patient but may be as high as 40 mg a day or as low as 5 mg a day. Thus the incidence of dangers and complications of long-term steroid therapy may be very high. Eventually the disease process may burn itself out and the patient can be weaned off steroids. Other immunosuppressive drugs, such as azathioprine and methotrexate have been tried in the management of pemphigus, but they are not as effective as steroids and are not without their own side effects. It would seem at present that they have little part to play in the treatment of this disease.

### Pemphigoid

Pemphigoid is the adjective form of the word pemphigus, and was originally used to mean pemphigus-like. Pemphigoid has now been split off from pemphigus on clinical, histological and immunological criteria.

Pemphigoid is most commonly seen in elderly patients. Unlike pemphigus the site of blister formation is at the basement membrane between the epidermis and dermis. Thus the roof of the blister is thicker and is less likely to rupture than in pemphigus. The patient therefore presents with fairly tense blisters varying in size from a few millimetres to a few centimetres in diameter (Figure 14.9). These may be widespread (Figure 14.10), and involve any part of the skin although the commonest sites are the limbs (Figure 14.11). Another clinical feature which is present in pemphigoid is large, confluent areas of skin which are erythematous and raised, giving plaque-like lesions. If these are present, it is usual to find the blisters in these red areas and not on normal looking skin (Figure 14.11). Mucosal lesions may occur, but are usually confined to the mouth, and are less frequent than in pemphigus. If untreated the disease will run a chronic course over a period of years and does not carry a high mortality like pemphigus.

### Aetiology

Pemphigoid, like pemphigus, is now considered to be one of the so-called auto-immune disorders. The antibody found in pemphigoid is different from that present in pemphigus, and is active against the basement membrane. The antibody

**Figure 14.9** *Blisters of varying size on the arm in pemphigoid.*

**Figure 14.10** *Widespread involvement in pemphigoid. A large number of blisters show signs of resolution.*

**Figure 14.11** *Erythematous, urticarial plaques in pemphigoid. The blisters tend to be found on these plaques.*

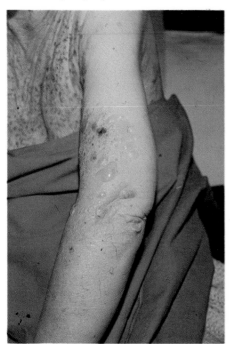
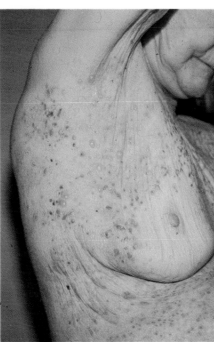
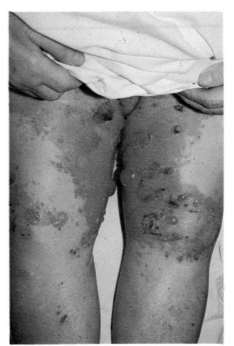

can be detected in the skin at the edge of the blisters and in the blood. Thus the antibody can be detected by immuno-fluorescent studies on the skin (direct) (Figure 14.12), or in the blood (indirect). The point should be stressed again that at present it is not certain whether the antibody is primary or secondary, but its detection has helped in the differential diagnosis of blistering eruptions.

### Treatment

The treatment of pemphigoid is with oral steroids. The initial dose is comparatively high, but not as high as that in pemphigus. It is usual to start with 60–80 mg of prednisone daily. As soon as new blisters stop appearing the dose of prednisone is gradually reduced. A maintenance dose of prednisone is usually necessary to control the disorder and is about 10–15 mg daily. There is some evidence that other immunosuppressive drugs, particularly azathioprine, are helpful in the maintenance treatment but not in the acute initial stages. Eventually the disease may burn itself out and the drugs can be stopped.

## Mucous Membrane Pemphigoid

This seems to be an entity separate from pemphigoid. The initial site of lesions may be any mucous membrane including the nose, larynx, pharynx, oesophagus, penis, vulva, vagina, anus and conjunctivae. The conjunctivae (Figure 14.13) are most frequently affected, being involved in 75 per cent of cases. The skin surrounding the body orifices may be affected, the lesions being tense sub-epidermal blisters as in ordinary pemphigoid. The distinctive feature of this disorder is that unlike pemphigus and pemphigoid it causes scarring of the affected areas.

### Treatment

Systemic corticosteroids are helpful in controlling the disease if it is extensive. If localised to a mucous membrane of only

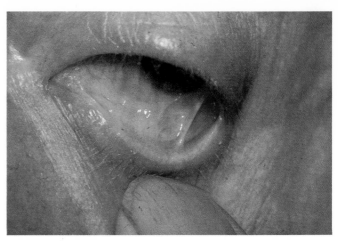

**Figure 14.13** *Scarring of the conjunctiva in 'mucous membrane' pemphigoid.*

**Figure 14.14**
*Grouped, excoriated lesions on knees in dermatitis herpetiformis.*

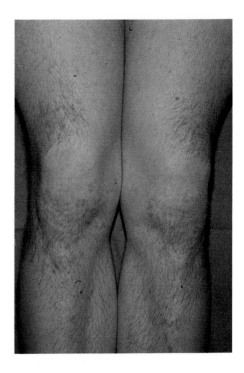

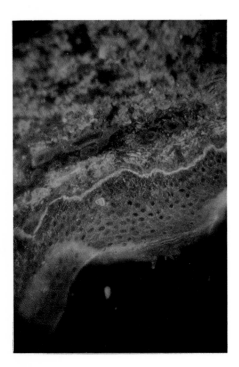

**Figure 14.12**
*Detection of pemphigoid antibody by immuno-fluorescence. A band of light green florescence is seen at the site of the basement membrane.*

**Figure 14.15** *Dermatitis herpetiformis. The elbows and extensor surface of the forearms are the commonest site of involvement.*

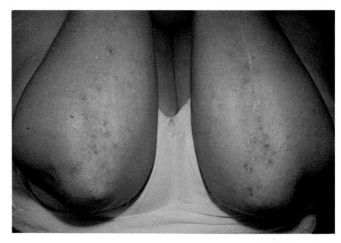

one organ then systemic treatment is not always justified. Subconjunctival injections of corticosteroid may be helpful in ocular involvement but neither these nor systemic steroids will always halt the progress of the disorder.

### Dermatitis Herpetiformis

The skin lesions of dermatitis herpetiformis may appear at any time in adult life, although the commonest age of presentation is in the third decade. The lesions occur most frequently on the knees (Figure 14.14), elbows (Figure 14.15 and 14.16), buttocks (Figure 14.17) and areas of pressure from clothing. However, the lesions may occur on any part of the skin, and the area over the scapulae is another common site (Figure 14.18).

The typical lesion is a small blister (Figures 14.16 and 14.19), and the lesions are often grouped (Figure 14.17), hence the term herpetiform. As in pemphigoid the blisters may occur on red, raised plaques of surrounding skin (Figures 14.17 and 14.19). The lesions are intensely irritating and because of this it is more frequent for the patient to present with an excoriated, papular eruption rather than blisters, the blisters having been destroyed by continual scratching (Figures 14.14, 14.15, 14.18 and 14.19). Dermatitis herpetiformis is a chronic and persistent disorder although occasionally there may be short remissions. The severity of the eruption varies considerably from patient to patient; in some the rash is generalised while in others it is confined to the elbows.

### Aetiology

All patients with dermatitis herpetiformis have a gluten sensitive enteropathy. However, in the majority of these patients this is subclinical and thus does not give rise to any symptoms, although on investigation there is a high incidence of folate and iron deficiency. The blister in dermatitis herpetiformis is subepidermal and the primary pathology in the skin occurs in the dermal papillae just *below* the basement membrane. It has now been established that in the *uninvolved* skin of patients with dermatitis herpetiformis there are deposits of immunoglobulins class A (IgA) on the reticulin fibres in the dermal papillae. IgA is the principal immunoglobulin produced by the gastro-intestinal tract and it is likely that an immune complex related to gluten is formed, and this is deposited on the reticulin fibres of the skin in dermatitis herpetiformis. Reticulin is involved in the disease process and anti-reticulin antibodies are detected in the blood. The detection of IgA deposits in the uninvolved skin is the simplest and most reliable test for establishing the diagnosis of dermatitis herpetiformis (Figure 14.20).

### Treatment

Ideally all patients with dermatitis herpetiformis should be investigated to assess the structural and functional state of their small intestine. The best treatment for dermatitis

**Figure 14.18** (Right) *Excoriated lesions over the shoulders, scapulae and centre of the back in dermatitis herpetiformis. Excoriations due to generalised non-specific irritation are only found over the upper shoulders.*

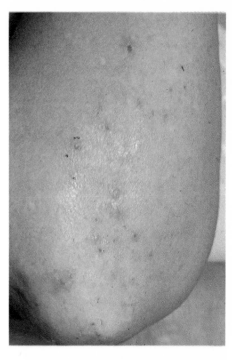

**Figure 14.16** *Small blisters and excoriated lesions on the elbow in dermatitis herpetiformis.*

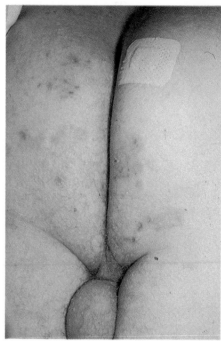

**Figure 14.17** *Grouped, urticarial and excoriated lesions on the buttocks in dermatitis herpetiformis.*

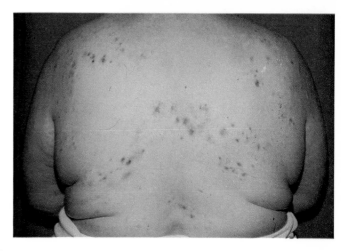

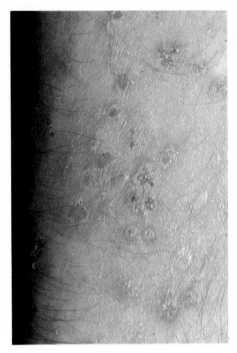

**Figure 14.19** *Blisters (some broken by scratching) on surrounding urticarial skin in dermatitis herpetiformis.*

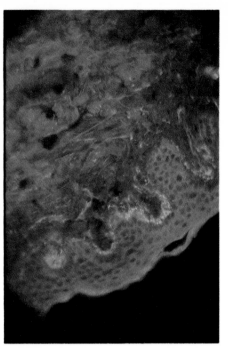

**Figure 14.20** *IgA deposits (fluorescing bright green) in the dermal papillae of the uninvolved skin in dermatitis herpetiformis.*

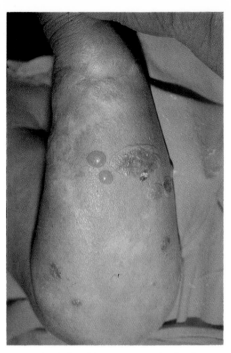

**Figure 14.21** *Herpes gestationis. Large, erythematous plaque with blisters.*

herpetiformis is a gluten-free diet as this treats both the intestinal and skin lesions. However, it must be stressed that it takes approximately one to two years of a gluten-free diet before the skin lesions disappear. This persistence must be related to the production of anti-reticulin antibody which continues for some time after gluten withdrawal. It must also be emphasised that the gluten-free diet must be strict, and it is a life-long treatment.

The skin lesions can be adequately controlled in the majority of patients by dapsone (approximately 100 mg daily). The mechanism of action of dapsone in dermatitis herpetiformis is not understood. However, the rash clears within a few days of commencing the drug, but it also re-appears within a few days of stopping it. Dapsone has no effect on the intestinal lesion. It causes haemolysis and in some patients this is severe, resulting in significant anaemia. For this reason patients taking dapsone for dermatitis herpetiformis should have frequent estimations of their haemoglobin concentration after initiating the drug, and when they are stabilised the haemoglobin concentration need be estimated only once a year. Dapsone causes methaemoglobinaemia in some patients. If patients are unable to tolerate this drug, sulphapyridine may be effective in controlling their lesions.

### Herpes Gestationis

This is an eruption occurring during pregnancy (usually after the fifth month) or early in the puerperium. The rash may be irritating like dermatitis herpetiformis but the distribution is not the same; it may effect any part of the skin. Herpes gestationis frequently begins with annular erythematous and urticarial lesions which subsequently may be associated

**Figure 14.22**
*Loss of toe-nails in epidermolysis bullosa.*

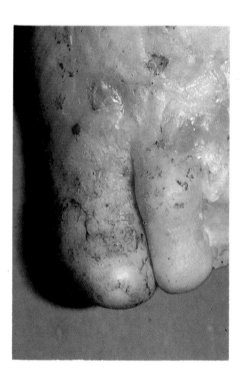

with blister formation. The blisters tend to be tense and may vary in diameter from a few millimetres to a few centimetres. The eruption has features similar to those of erythema multiforme and pemphigoid (Figure 14.21). The eruption usually responds to systemic corticosteroids, at a dose of 20–30 mg prednisone per day. The skin lesions will clear and not require further treatment after the end of the puerperium. The exact cause of the disorder is unknown but there is evidence for an immunological basis for the rash.

Complement is found to the basement membrane as in pemphigoid and in a number of patients an antibody to the basement membrane has been detected. It would appear that pregnancy in some way alters the immunological status of the individual, for the rash clears after delivery, but frequently returns in subsequent pregnancies.

## Epidermolysis Bullosa

This rather cumbersome name is used to describe a group of congenital blistering disorders. All the syndromes are genetically determined. In the simple form there is spontaneous blister formation on the hands and feet from birth and later in life at the sites of even slight trauma of the skin. In this form the blisters heal leaving no scars. In the more severe forms there may be scarring and subsequent contractural deformity of the hands and feet. The teeth and nails (Figure 14.22) may also be abnormal in certain forms of epidermolysis bullosa. In the severe forms there may be involvement of the mucous membranes of the mouth, pharynx, and oesophagus; the most serious complication being oesophageal stricture.

### Treatment

In the simple form no treatment is usually required, although topical steroids sometimes shorten the duration of the blisters. In the more severe forms the disorder can be helped by systemic steroids, but any benefit has to be weighed against the complications of long-term steroid therapy.

# 15. Malignant Conditions of the Skin

## Basal Cell Epithelioma

THIS is sometimes referred to as a basal cell carcinoma or by its common name of 'rodent ulcer'. Basal cell epithelioma is the commonest malignant tumour of the skin. It usually occurs on the face, the commonest site being below the eyes or the sides of the nose (Figure 15.1). Basal cell epithelioma appears to be induced by ultra-violet light as the condition is much commoner in countries like South Africa and Australia. The degree of pigmentation of the skin is also an important factor, the tumour being more frequent in fair skinned people and rarely developing in negroes. Basal cell epithelioma is also sometimes seen in the skin many years after radiotherapy for non-malignant conditions, e.g. tinea capitis, but fortunately the use of radiotherapy for non-malignant skin conditions is now, or should be, a thing of the past. Multiple basal cell epitheliomata, usually on the trunk, are seen many years after prolonged arsenic therapy (Figure 15.2), but again this fortunately is becoming rare. It may take thirty to forty years for basal cell epitheliomata to appear after radiotherapy or arsenic.

Basal cell epithelioma is usually a condition of middle-aged and elderly persons, but very rarely may be seen in younger people usually of European descent who have lived in countries which have a great deal of strong sunshine. It may occur in children or teenagers as part of a genetically determined disorder associated with skeletal abnormalities.

### Clinical Presentations

1. *Ulcer.* The commonest morphology is for the lesion to begin as a small papule which then spreads outwards, leaving a central ulcer (Figure 15.1). Telangiectasia may be seen in the raised and pearl-coloured edges which are characteristic of basal cell epithelioma (Figures 15.3 and 15.4). Once the lesion ulcerates it bleeds and patients often present with a 'persistent scab' which fails to heal (Figures

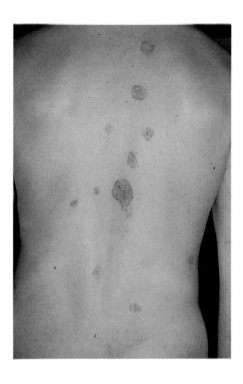

**Figure 15.2** *Multiple basal cell epitheliomata on the trunk following arsenic taken for psoriasis thirty years previously.*

**Figure 15.1** *The commonest sites for basal cell epitheliomata are below the eyes and the sides of the nose.*

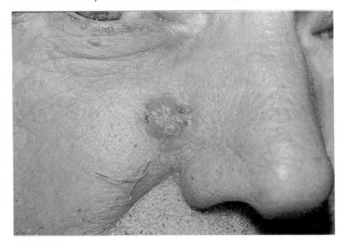

**Figure 15.3** *Basal cell epithelioma with raised, pearly edges. Telangiectasia is visible in the edges and ulceration is beginning in the centre.*

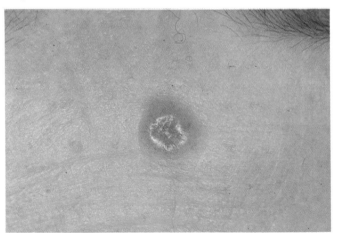

15.5 and 15.6). If this is the case the edges should be carefully examined to see if they are raised and pearly (Figures 15.5 and 15.6). If in doubt the scab should be removed with a pair of forceps. If left untreated the lesion will spread over the skin in an annular fashion and inwards to involve the underlying structures.

2. *Cystic type*. Occasionally there is no ulceration but continuous enlargement and the presenting feature is then a cystic pearl-coloured lesion (Figures 15.7 and 15.8) with an irregular surface but no ulcer. Telangiectasia can usually be seen on the surface.

3. *Morphoeic type*. This is a relatively rare form, but can present diagnostic difficulties if it is not known. The presenting feature is a firm white plaque, usually on the face. There may or may not be ulceration. This type of lesion is due to a fibrotic reaction to the carcinoma with an attempt at healing. It is very slow-growing and persistent. Occasional scarring in a basal cell epithelioma may be seen. Features of the original lesion are still visible (Figure 15.9) and in these instances the diagnosis should be easier.

4. *Pigmented type*. Occasionally the cystic form or the 'clas-sical ulcer' becomes pigmented (Figure 15.10). In these circumstances it may be difficult to distinguish the lesion from a malignant melanoma, particularly if the whole structure is pigmented.

5. *Superficial type*. This is a form of basal carcinoma usually seen on the trunk (Figure 15.2). It is relatively rare. The lesion tends not to be invasive (hence the name) and spreads on the surface in all directions. The patient usually presents with a discoid erythematous lesion which may have small ulcers in it and a raised pearly edge (Figure 15.11).

## Prognosis

The prognosis of a basal cell carcinoma is usually excellent, because it does not metastasise and is very slow-growing. Thus if the patient seeks advice early on there should be a complete cure. If the lesions are left untreated they may prove fatal after many years as they will erode deeper structures, and are then often untreatable.

## Treatment

1. *Radiotherapy*. Before radiotherapy the lesion should be

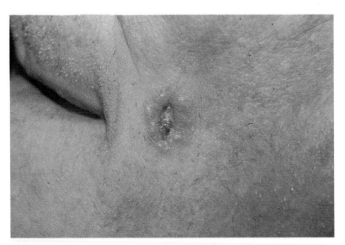

**Figure 15.4** *Typical basal cell epithelioma. The lesion shows central ulceration and raised pearly edges with telangiectasia.*

**Figure 15.5** *Basal cell epithelioma presenting as a persistent scab on the nose. The edges are slightly raised and one edge is pearly with telangiectasia.*

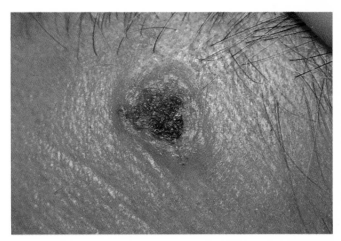

**Figure 15.6** *Persistent scab on the forehead surrounded by raised edges. This is a common presentation of a basal cell epithelioma.*

**Figure 15.7** *Cystic type of basal cell epithelioma. Raised 'pearly' lesion with telangiectasia.*

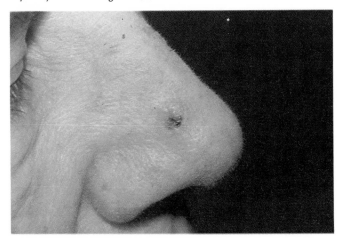

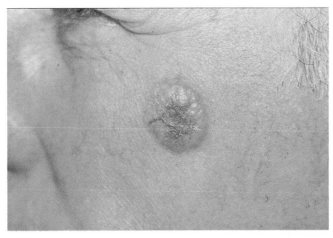

biopsied to confirm the clinical diagnosis. If radiotherapy is carried out in a good centre then the cure rate is of the order of 95 per cent. This treatment is simple and is probably the treatment of choice for elderly patients. However, when dealing with younger persons it should be remembered that radiotherapy given in a therapeutic dose for carcinoma will probably produce scarring and telangiectasia in the site five to ten years later.

2. *Surgery*. Excision is the treatment of choice in younger persons and also offers a cure rate of 95 per cent in the right hands.

3. *Curettage and Cautery*. For lesions less than 1 cm in diameter it has been shown that a 90 per cent cure rate can be produced using this type of treatment. Although the recurrence rate is higher than with surgery or radiotherapy, the cosmetic result with small lesions may be better.

4. *Topical cytotoxic drugs*. These have been tried in recent years, the most successful being 5-fluorouracil or podophyllin extracts. However, the place for this treatment in routine cases has not yet been established although promising results have been obtained in the superficial type.

## Squamous Cell Epithelioma

The common sites for squamous cell epitheliomata are the exposed areas of skin, lips and tongue. Skin on the back of

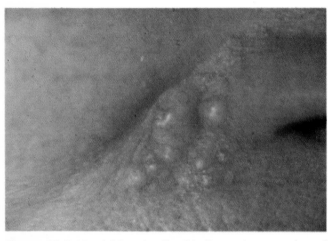

**Figure 15.8** *'Cystic' basal cell epithelioma. A group of pearl coloured lesions with no ulceration.*

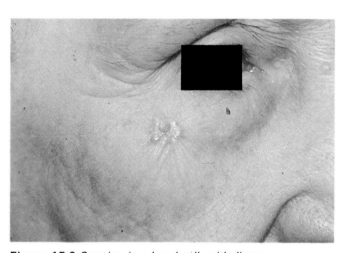

**Figure 15.9** *Scarring in a basal cell epithelioma.*

**Figure 15.11** *'Superficial' type of basal cell epithelioma usually found on the trunk. The lesion progresses along the surface of the skin but is not usually invasive. The lesion is usually a red, scaly plaque with a raised pearly edge.*

**Figure 15.10** *Melanin pigmentation beginning in a basal cell epithelioma.*

**Figure 15.12** *Squamous cell epithelioma on the back of the hand. The lesion presented as a nodule with a small central scab.*

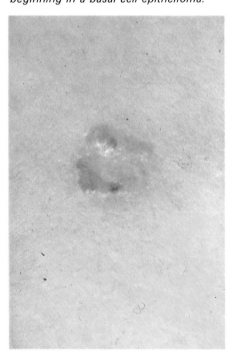

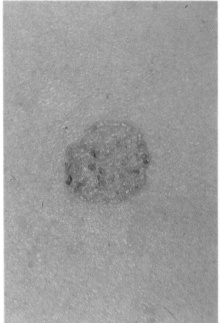

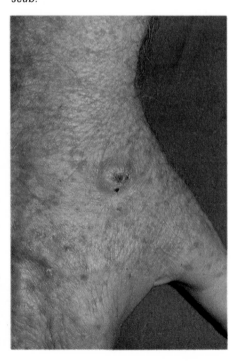

**Figure 15.14** (Right) *Squamous cell epithelioma on the lip presenting as a hyperkeratotic tumour. The lesion began in chronically inflamed skin affected by discoid lupus erythematosus.*

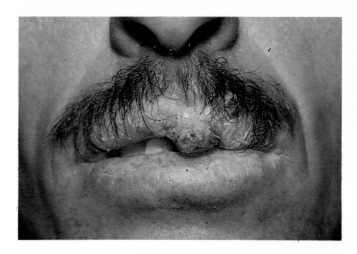

the hands (Figures 15.12 and 15.13), pinnae, and lips (Figures 15.14 and 15.15) appear to be particularly prone to develop squamous cell epitheliomata. Because the lesions are more common on the exposed than the unexposed skin, sunlight has been incriminated in the causation of these lesions as with basal cell epitheliomata. However, squamous cell lesions are common on the lips and back of the hands, and these are extremely rare sites for basal cell lesions. Squamous cell epitheliomata also occur at sites of chronic trauma, and of some chronic skin disorders, e.g. discoid lupus erythematosus (Figure 15.14).

### Clinical Features

The epithelioma begins as a small nodule which grows to form an oval or circular tumour (Figures 15.12 and 15.14). The lesion may break down and present as an ulcer (Figure 15.13), usually, but not always, with rolled edges. It may alternatively present as a scabbed nodule (Figure 15.12). On the lip it may present as a small *persistent* fissure or ulcer (Figure 15.15) and such lesions should be biopsied.

### Prognosis

Although this type of carcinoma has an excellent prognosis compared to carcinomata involving internal organs, it does not have such a good prognosis as the basal cell epithelioma. The squamous cell lesion has the ability to metastasise. However, if it is treated early the prognosis is good.

### Treatment

The diagnosis should be established by biopsy, and treatment is then by surgery or radiotherapy, or both.

### Keratoacanthoma

Although this lesion is not malignant it is convenient to discuss it here because it is often the differential diagnosis

**Figure 15.15**
*Squamous cell epithelioma presenting as a small persistent ulcer on the lower lip.*

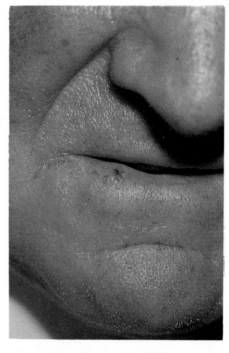

**Figure 15.13** *Squamous cell epithelioma presenting as a persistent ulcer on the back of the hand.*

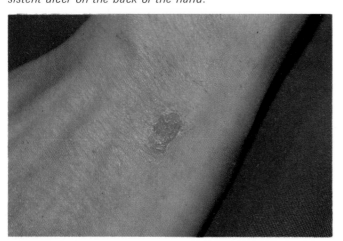

**Figure 15.16**
*Keratoacanthoma. Raised lesion with central keratin plug.*

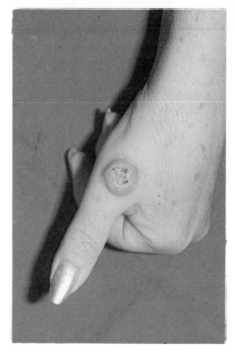

95

when considering basal and squamous cell carcinomata.

Keratoacanthoma is not uncommon, and presents as a small papule which rapidly grows in size over a period of three months. The lesion is often raised 0.5 cm above the surrounding skin surface and is usually 1 to 2 cm in diameter. The edges are rolled and there is a central depression with a thickened keratin plug (Figure 15.16). If this becomes detached the lesion may well be similar to an ulcerating epithelioma. If left untreated the keratoacanthoma would maintain the size it had achieved after its three-month growing period for a further three months and then involute after another three months.

### Treatment

Because of the differential diagnosis it is important that keratoacanthomata are biopsied to establish the correct diagnosis. Once this has been done it would be in order to leave the lesion alone and await its spontaneous resolution. However, because the commonest site is the face, the patient often asks for treatment. If the lesion is a centimetre or less in diameter then curettage and cautery is the simplest treatment. With larger lesions radiotherapy will be necessary. The cause of keratoacanthomata is as yet unknown.

### Malignant Melanoma

This is a relatively rare tumour when compared to basal cell carcinomata. The malignant melanoma may occur anywhere on the skin surface, but the legs have a relatively higher incidence than other parts of the body.

Malignant melanomata do *not* always arise in pre-existing

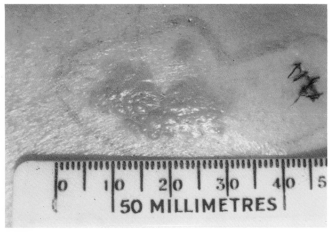

**Figure 15.17** *Amelanotic malignant melanoma with satellite lesions.*

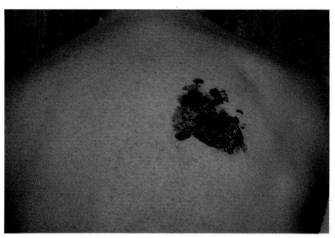

**Figure 15.19** *Large pigmented malignant melanoma with satellite lesions. The lesion has an irregular surface, and there is variation in the degree of pigmentation.*

**Figure 15.18** *Large ulcerated amelanotic melanoma.*

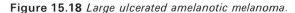

**Figure 15.20** *Malignant melanoma. Pigmented nodule and area of surrounding pigmentation.*

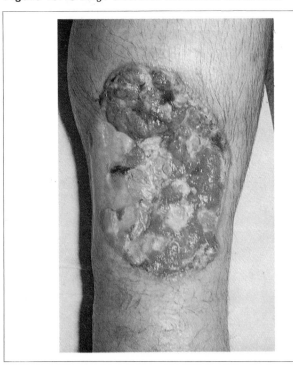

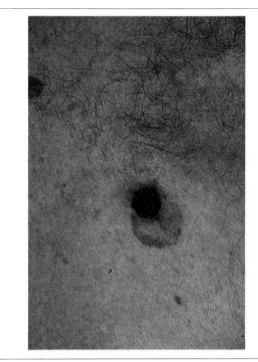

'moles' or pigmented naevi, and it is not known what percentage arise from moles and what percentage at sites where there was no preceding lesion.

### Clinical Features

The lesion is usually but *not always* pigmented (Figures 15.17 and 15.18). If any of the following features are reported then malignant melanoma should be suspected:

(a) Increase in size of a pigmented lesion. There may also be satellite pigmented lesions (Figure 15.19).

(b) Alteration in pigmentation of the lesion. The skin surrounding the lesion may also show alteration of pigmentation, either increased (Figure 15.20) or decreased (Figure 15.21).

(c) Ulceration or bleeding of a pigmented or non-pigmented lesion (Figure 15.18).

### Prognosis

Although the prognosis of malignant melanoma is usually thought to be poor, this is not always so, though what influences the ultimate prognosis is unknown. The story of the patient who has the lesion excised and dies thirty years later from widespread secondary deposits is well known, and a similar lesion treated in the same way may kill the patient in a matter of weeks.

### Treatment

This is usually by surgery with wide excision and skin graft.

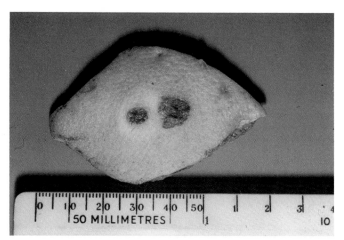

**Figure 15.21** *Malignant melanoma. Two pigmented lesions, one showing an area of depigmentation.*

**Figure 15.22** *Bowen's disease (intra-epidermal carcinoma). Localised and persistent red, scaly lesion.*

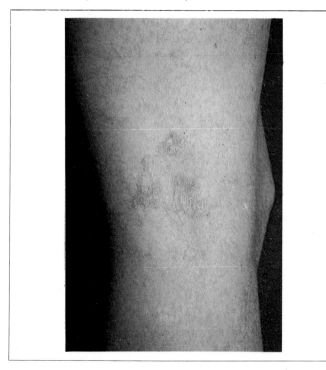

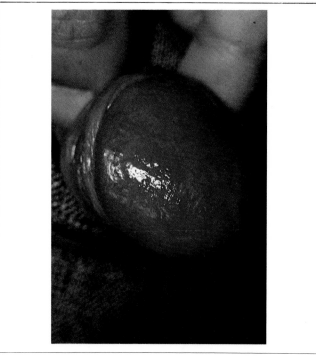

**Figure 15.23** *Erythroplasia of Queyrat. Persistent red, moist area, with a 'velvety' appearance, on the glans penis.*

**Figure 15.24** *Paget's disease of the breast.*

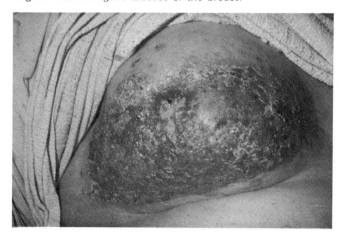

97

Treatment of secondary deposits will vary for each particular case. For very widespread disease immunotherapy is now being used. Radiotherapy is also sometimes used for treatment of the primary lesions.

## Intra-epidermal Epithelioma

### Bowen's Disease

This is a carcinoma *in situ*. The lesion is confined to the epidermis and may not become invasive for many years. It is, however, potentially malignant and may change to a squamous cell epithelioma.

It may involve any part of the skin. The lesion usually presents as a solitary reddish brown scaly plaque (Figure 15.22). The edges may be slightly raised with papillomatous growth. It is very slow-growing but persistent.

#### *Treatment*

The diagnosis should be established by biopsy. If the lesion is small it can be removed by curettage and cautery or excision; if it is over 2 cm in diameter a graft will probably be necessary after surgery. Radiotherapy or topical 5-fluoro uracil may also be used.

### Erythroplasia of Queyrat

This is the name given to intra-epidermal carcinoma of the glans penis (Figure 15.23). The lesion presents as a persistent red, moist area with a 'velvety' appearance.

#### *Treatment*

The treatment of choice is topical 5-fluorouracil. This is usually successful and radiotherapy and surgery are not necessary.

### Paget's Disease

This is also an intra-epidermal carcinoma. The commonest site is the nipple and areola of the female breast in the middle aged. It usually presents as unilateral erythema and scaling, and looks eczematous (Figure 15.24). In the later stages there may be destruction of the nipple. Unfortunately, the condition is usually part of an intra-ductal carcinoma and treatment therefore is mastectomy.

## Senile or Actinic Keratoses

These lesions are not themselves malignant but may eventually turn into squamous cell epitheliomata. As the name implies they are found in the areas exposed to light, and are commoner in fair people and those living in climates which have a great deal of sunshine.

The lesions are discrete and raised with a 'crumbling' surface (Figure 15.25). They have a greyish brown appearance and are usually numerous. There are usually other signs of excessive exposure to ultra-violet light, such as pigmented patches and thinning of the skin. The top of the lesion may be knocked off by trauma and leave a small superficial ulcer.

## Treatment

The lesions are purely epidermal and may be treated with

**Figure 15.25**
*Actinic keratosis.
Greyish-brown
scaly lesion.*

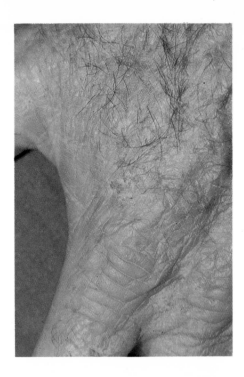

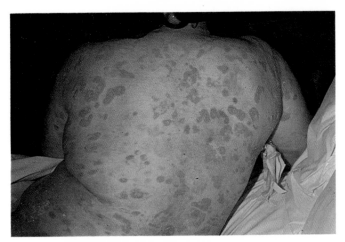

**Figure 15.26** *Mycosis fungoides, presenting as persistent red, scaly patches, which may be mistaken for eczema or psoriasis in the early stages.*

**Figure 15.27** *Ulcerating infiltrated tumour in mycosis fungoides.*

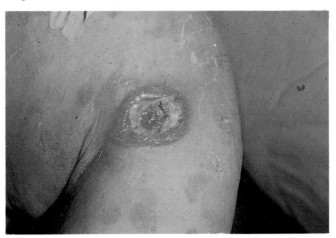

cryotherapy or electrocautery. If the lesions are numerous the best treatment is topical 5-fluorouracil.


## Skin Reticulosis

*Mycosis fungoides*. This is a distinctive reticulosis as it originates in the skin and continues predominantly as a skin disorder, but may eventually be associated with a reticulosis involving internal organs.

It is rare in childhood but may begin in early adult life or subsequently at any age. In the early stages the disease presents as persistent erythematous scaly patches (Figure 15.26) on any part of the skin, and may look like eczema or psoriasis. The lesions may persist in this form for many years before becoming infiltrated nodules which eventually ulcerate (Figure 15.27). Although the disease is invariably fatal the whole course may be over many years, and elderly patients frequently die from other causes.

## Treatment

In the early stages the lesions may be controlled to a certain extent by the powerful topical corticosteroids. These drugs can certainly suppress the accompanying inflammatory reaction in the skin and may be helpful in alleviating any irritation. In the later stages radiotherapy is effective in controlling the lesions if they are not too widespread. If the disease is very extensive total body electron beam therapy often produces a remission. There have been favourable reports of the efficacy of photochemotherapy (psoralens with long wave ultra-violet light), although current cytotoxic drugs do not appear to be very effective in controlling the disease.

## Other Reticuloses

Sarcomata, leukaemia, and Hodgkin's disease may appear as infiltrated papules or plaques in the skin which occasionally are the presenting feature of these disorders. The diagnosis is established by biopsy.

# 16. Acne and Rosacea

## Acne

Acne is now used synonymously with, and has virtually replaced, the term acne vulgaris. Acne is essentially a disorder of adolescence, and it has been estimated that up to 80 per cent of all adolescents will have some degree of acne varying from a few comedones to severe cystic lesions. The commonest age of onset is at puberty but acne may appear a year or two before. However, it should also be appreciated that acne may begin after puberty and even in persons (particularly females) in the third and fourth decades. The natural history is variable. The disorder may last only a few months in the mildest forms but usually it will persist from puberty to the late teens or early twenties. In some patients the acne will persist into adult life even until middle age although the severity of the disease will probably be less. It is not possible to predict at what age it will resolve, and caution should be exercised in telling patients they will grow out of it!

### Pathology

Acne is a disease which affects the pilo-sebaceous unit. The primary defect appears to be excess keratin production at the opening of the pilo-sebaceous unit which prevents the escape of sebum. A comedone (blackhead) subsequently forms; this is a mass of keratin and sebum. The upper portion of the blackhead is darkened by melanin from melanocytes in the adjacent epidermis, the lower part of the comedo remains a yellowish white colour. Comedones as described above are sometimes referred to as 'open'; or they may be 'closed', i.e. not reaching the surface of the skin to be extruded. In the latter instances the sebaceous gland continues to produce sebum and the gland begins to swell and eventually ruptures intradermally. In these circumstances the sebum which escapes into the dermis is an irritant and therefore sets up a foreign body reaction. Thus there is erythema and pus formation, and the area tends to be 'walled off' by the connective tissue cells, and healing occurs with subsequent fibrosis. The degree of the inflammation and subsequent scarring varies greatly between patients even if the sebaceous glands rupture and may well depend on the composition of sebum, and on how irritant the sebum is to the surrounding tissues. In some instances of severe inflammation cyst formation occurs, the so-called acne cyst. It should be stressed that the pathology of acne does not appear to be initiated or continued by bacteria.

### Aetiology

The basic causes of acne are not yet known but undoubtedly it is in some way related to hormones because of the onset at or about the time of puberty and the fact that acne is often worse pre-menstrually. However it appears that an 'end organ effect' rather than the circulating levels of the hormones are the cause of acne.

**Figure 16.1** *Acne on the face, the commonest site.*

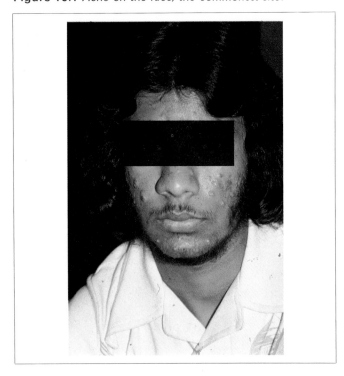

**Figure 16.2** *Resolving acne on the chest. It is usually the centre and upper regions of the chest that are involved.*

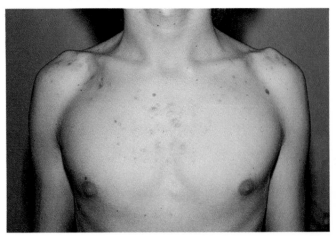

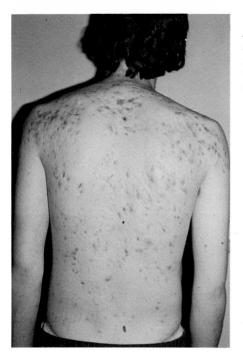

## Clinical Features

*Sites.* Acne lesions occur on the face, centre of the chest, back above the waistline, shoulders and occasionally neck (Figures 16.1, 16.2 and 16.3). These tend to be the areas which have more sebaceous glands per unit surface area than other parts of the skin. The lesions may occur only on the face or only on parts of the face, i.e. forehead, cheeks, or along the chin, and the trunk is spared. Conversely, the lesions may occur only on the trunk with no involvement of the face. The back is more commonly affected than chest, and usually more severely.

*Types of lesion.* The initial lesion is the comedone or blackhead (Figure 16.4). If the comedones are closed then the gland ruptures and depending on the degree of inflammation the clinical appearance varies. If the inflammatory reaction is not severe a red papule forms (Figures 16.5 and 16.6); in more severe inflammatory reactions clinically visible pustules appear (Figures 16.6 and 16.7). Finally, cyst formation may occur (Figures 16.7, 16.8 and 16.9), the cysts being up to 2 cm in diameter. Because of the inflammation,

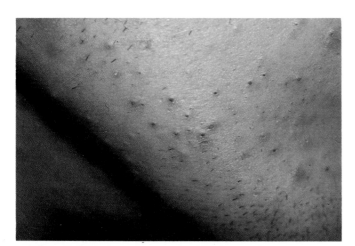

**Figure 16.4** *Comedones or blackheads, the primary lesion in acne.*

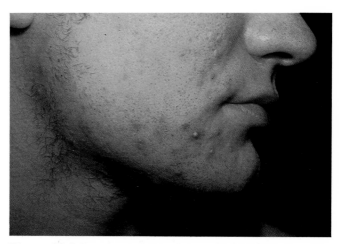

**Figure 16.6** *Papules and pustules on the face in acne.*

**Figure 16.5** *Erythematous papules on the face in acne.*

**Figure 16.7** *Comedones, papules, pustules and cysts, the four types of lesion found in acne.*

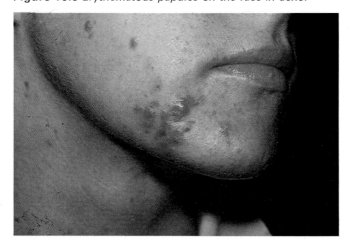

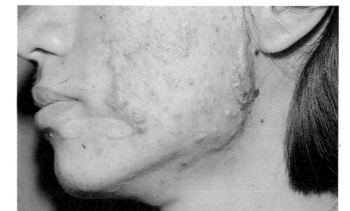

the skin surrounding the lesions is red compared to the uninvolved skin. If the inflammatory response has been severe, there is fibrosis and scarring, the scars often appearing as small, depressed pits (Figure 16.10). Occasionally, as with other scars, keloid formation may occur (Figure 16.11). It should be stressed that just as the sites of involvement vary between patients so may the types of lesion, i.e. some patients have only comedones, whilst others have only papules and pustules, and some have only cysts. Alternatively, there may be patients with all types of lesions. The reasons for this variation are not known.

## Management and Treatment

A large number of people do not seek treatment for their acne, and know that the disorder has no internal consequences. However, because the lesions are unsightly and most frequently occur during adolescence many do ask for help. It appears that the patient's personality is important in deciding whether to ask for medical advice. If patients do ask for treatment the worst possible approach is to tell them they will grow out of their troubles by the time they are twenty-one and to do nothing for them.

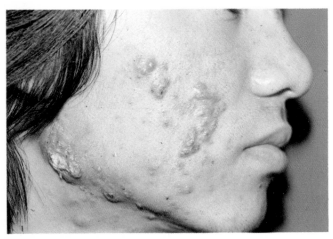

**Figure 16.8** *Cystic acne. One of the lesions has been discharging and has now scabbed.*

**Figure 16.9** *Cysts on the neck in acne.*

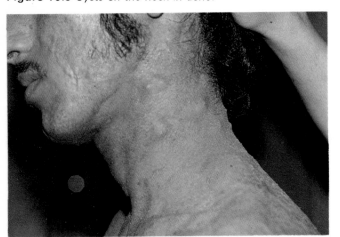

### General Measures

*Diet*. In the past great emphasis has been placed on diet, and patients have been advised to cut out chocolates, sweets and fatty meats and to reduce their fat and/or carbohydrate intake depending on what is 'fashionable' at that particular time. However, there is no worthwhile evidence as yet to show that manipulation of the diet has a part to play in the management of acne.

*Cleansing*. It is often implied that patients with acne do not wash frequently enough. Although frequent washing with soap and water may help slightly by removing excess keratin and sebum and thus decrease comedone formation, lack of washing with soap and water does not cause acne. Because acne is not primarily an infective condition, antiseptic soaps and lotions are not indicated.

*Debridement*. Removal of large comedones produces definite cosmetic improvement and is sometimes helpful in preventing superficial pustulation. It will not have any effect on deeper inflammatory lesions. Comedones should be removed, after soaking the area with a hot towel for a few minutes, by a comedone extractor. Incision of lesions is not helpful and will leave scars.

*Sunlight*. Ultra-violet light is often beneficial in acne, probably due to the 'peeling effect' it has on the skin which prevents blockage of the pilo-sebaceous units. In summer, patients should be instructed to be in the sun when practical and artificial ultra-violet light may be given in some cases if benefit is derived. Occasionally some patients appear to be made worse by ultra-violet light, but this is more often due to heat and humidity which causes swelling of the keratin and further blockage of the pilo-sebaceous units.

*Topical measures*. Any substance which breaks up keratin may unblock the pilo-sebaceous unit and allow drainage of the sebum. One to 5 per cent of sulphur, salicylic acid or resorcinol, either in spirit or a cream base, have all been used in the past and may have a beneficial effect on acne. These preparations should be applied at night. It is ad-

**Figure 16.10** *Scarring due to acne. The scar on the face in acne is a 'small, depressed pit'.*

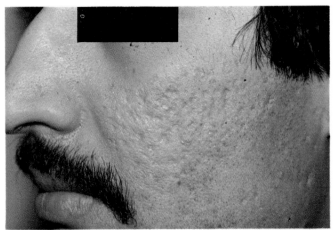

visable to start with one per cent of the preparation and increase the strength if the patient can tolerate it without making the skin too sore. More recently benzoyl peroxide has been used in proprietary preparations and these are also effective in some cases. Most topical preparations are useful only for comedones and superficial papules and pustules.

*Systemic therapy.* Tetracyclines appear to be of benefit in a large proportion of patients with acne in whom there is inflammation with papules and pustules. The mechanism of action of tetracyclines is as yet unknown, although it does not appear to be due to its anti-bacterial properties. If tetracycline is to be prescribed the commencing dose should be 250 mg b.d. for at least six weeks. After this time the dose may be titrated against the activity of the condition. Many patients can be kept free of their acne on a maintenance dose of 250 mg on alternate days. Patients should always be advised to tail off the tetracycline slowly, and not stop suddenly. If there is no improvement after three months on tetracyclines, then other antibiotics should be tried. There is as yet no rational explanation for the effectiveness of individual antibiotics in acne, and selection is therefore empirical. Other antibiotics which have been found to be effective in acne include cotrimoxazole, erythromycin and clindamycin. The regime is similar to that used for the tetracyclines, i.e. they are used for six to eight weeks, in a comparatively small dose, before any assessment is made. Maintenance treatment may have to be continued for many months or years in some patients to control the eruption.

Oestrogens are also effective in suppressing acne, and may be given to female patients. The best method of administration of oestrogens is as a high dose oestrogen contraceptive pill.

*Intra-lesional therapy.* The most effective way of treating acne cysts is with intra-lesional triamcinolone. This appears to counteract the inflammation and prevents scarring.

*Infantile acne.* Very occasionally typical acne lesions may

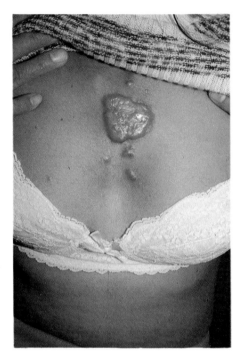

**Figure 16.11**
*Keloid formation on the chest due to acne lesions.*

**Figure 16.12** *Mild rosacea affecting only the nose and cheeks. There is erythema and telangiectasia.*

**Figure 16.13** *Persistent erythema of the face in rosacea.*

**Figure 16.14** *Erythematous, papular eruption on the chin, cheeks and forehead in rosacea. The skin surrounding the papules is erythematous.*

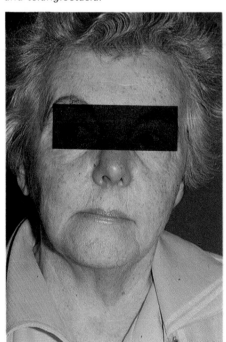

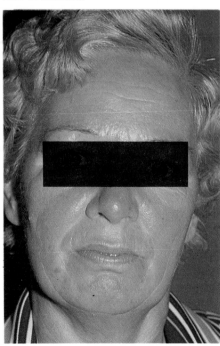

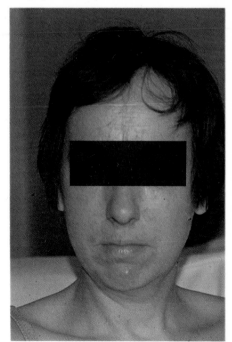

103

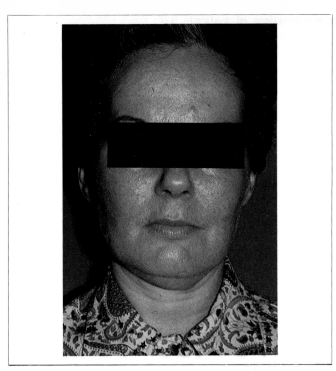

**Figure 16.15** *Rosacea treated with topical steroids. The general erythema may be improved, but telangiectasia and papules persist and may be aggravated.*

appear on the cheeks of infants during the first few months of life and then subside. This is probably the effect of maternal hormones.

### Rosacea

This is a disorder of young and middle aged adults. Although the cause is unknown it appears to be a disorder of the blood vessels of the skin of the face. Rosacea only affects the face. It may affect all the face or only parts of it. The characteristic lesions are erythema, papules, pustules and telangiectasia. The erythema and telangiectasia may affect only the cheeks and nose (Figure 16.12), and the papules and pustules may occur only on the cheeks, forehead or chin. All or some of these areas may be involved. In the early stages there may be an exaggerated flushing of the skin in response to heat, to certain types of food or to emotional stress. Subsequently this erythema persists (Figure 16.13), and telangiectasia begins to appear. The next stage is the development of papules and pustules (Figure 16.14).

A variation of rosacea is rhinophyma. This is thickening of the skin of the nose, with associated gross hypertrophy of the sebaceous glands. It is usually the lower third of the nose which enlarges as a hyperaemic lobulated mass of tissue, pitted by the orifices of the sebaceous glands.

Ocular involvement may occur in rosacea. This usually takes the form of rosacea keratitis. The patient may initially complain of sore eyes, but subsequently pain and photophobia develop. In addition to the keratitis there may be blepharitis, conjunctivitis, iritis and even episcleritis. If not treated the keratitis may lead to ulceration and corneal opacities.

The natural history of rosacea is variable but it tends to be a chronic disorder persisting for a number of years.

### Treatment

#### *General Advice*

In the past it was often assumed that patients with rosacea also had chronic gastritis and for this reason they were told to omit alcohol, spicy food, strong tea and coffee. The benefit obtained from cutting down on these substances probably occurs because they tend to cause reflex vasodilatation of the skin blood vessels of the face. There is no evidence that patients with rosacea do in fact have gastritis.

#### *Topical Measures*

Sulphur in the strength of 1–2 per cent in a suitable cream base often helps when there are papules and pustules. Because steroids are the modern panacea of present day dermatology, patients with rosacea invariably receive these preparations. Initially they have a beneficial effect, probably because of their vasoconstrictor and anti-inflammatory actions, so that initially there is lessening of the erythema and decrease in the severity of papule and pustule formation. However, because rosacea may persist for years and steroids are only suppressive and not curative, they are probably best avoided, for if they are continued for any length of time, i.e. longer than a few months, there is atrophy of the underlying collagen and telangiectasia already present in rosacea becomes more prominent (Figure 16.15). In addition, when the topical steroids are stopped there is often a rebound phenomenon with exacerbation of the rosacea and pustule formation.

#### *Systemic Therapy*

The most effective treatment at the present time for rosacea is the tetracyclines. As with acne, their mechanism of action is not understood. The tetracyclines are prescribed in a régime similar to that for acne, usually 250 mg b.d. for at least six weeks, and the dose is then titrated against the activity of the disease process. Many patients can be controlled on a dose as low as 250 mg tetracycline twice weekly, but they find that if they stop the drug there is a relapse of the condition.

The eye complications of rosacea are best cared for by an ophthalmologist because of their potentially serious sequelae, but they too are often helped by systemic tetracyclines.

# 17. Lupus Erythematosus, Scleroderma and Dermatomyositis

THESE three diseases come into the group of *collagen disorders*. The diseases to be considered in this chapter have specific cutaneous manifestations, although there may also be systemic involvement.

## Lupus Erythematosus

There are two diseases which carry this name, the so-called 'chronic discoid' form and the 'acute systemic' variety. It is still uncertain whether there is a direct relationship between them (other than their name). Some authorities consider that on occasions the chronic form may pass into the systemic form, whilst others maintain they are two entirely separate diseases.

### Chronic Discoid Lupus Erythematosus

This disorder affects men and women equally, and usually commences in early or middle adult life. It tends to be a chronic disease lasting many years but the natural history has been altered in the last decade as it is now more readily controlled with the powerful topical corticosteroids.

### Sites of Involvement

The commonest site of involvement is the face (Figure 17.1), and the disorder frequently appears for the first time after exposure to sunlight. Lesions may also appear on the scalp, ears, neck (Figure 17.2), hands (Figure 17.3) and very occasionally on the arms and upper trunk. The lesions may be solitary, few in number or numerous and, even in the last instance, they tend not to be symmetrical.

### Morphology

In the early stages the lesion is a well-defined red plaque (Figures 17.1 and 17.3). The surface is scaly (Figures 17.2 and 17.3) and there is follicular dilatation. The scale extends into the follicles and if the scale from a lesion is removed in one piece, the follicular scales appear as small prominent

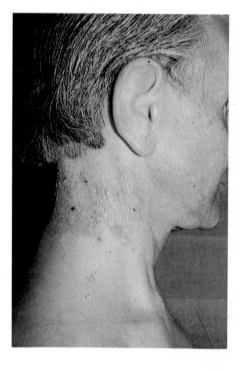

**Figure 17.2** *Red, scaly lesions of discoid lupus erythematosus on the neck after exposure to sunlight.*

**Figure 17.1** *Red, infiltrated patches of discoid lupus erythematosus on the cheeks. This is an early stage of the disorder.*

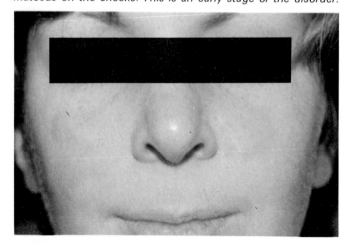

**Figure 17.3** *Plaques of discoid lupus erythematosus. The lesion has a scaly surface and follicular plugging is present.*

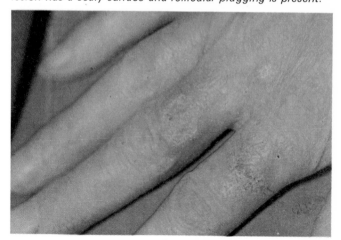

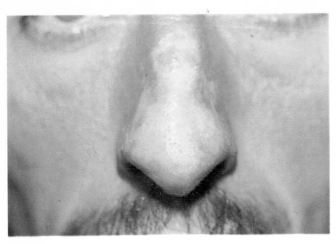

**Figure 17.4** *Atrophic plaque of discoid lupus erythematosus with follicular plugging.*

spines on the undersurface. However, if the superficial scale has been shed but the keratin remains in the hair follicles, the dilated follicles give the appearance of being 'plugged' with keratin (Figures 17.3 and 17.4). The size of the plaque is variable; it may be as small as 0.5 cm but is commonly 2 to 3 cm in diameter. Occasionally the lesions merge to form a large confluent plaque involving the entire forehead or a cheek. As the disease progresses there is scarring (Figure 17.5) and atrophic change in the skin, and telangiectasia and pigmentary changes may occur. Occasionally the lesions break down and ulcerate, and very rarely after many years may progress to a squamous cell carcinoma.

The mouth (Figure 17.6) or vagina are sometimes involved. At these sites the lesions appear as persistent erosions.

If the scalp is involved there will eventually be hair loss as there is destruction of the hair follicles (Figures 17.7 and 17.8).

In the end stages of the disorder when the disease process is 'burnt out' the site of involvement appears as white thickened scar tissue. It is not uncommon to see the disease still active in the periphery of a lesion while the centre is inactive, thus giving rise to a red annular scaly lesion with a white atrophic centre.

### Treatment

As has already been mentioned, discoid lupus erythematosus is adversely affected by sunlight, and thus patients should avoid exposure as much as possible. Sun barrier preparations should be used for lesions on the head and neck prior to patients going outdoors in the summer months.

*Topical steroids.* The powerful topical corticosteroids have improved the treatment and management of chronic discoid lupus erythematosus. Many lesions will respond to twice daily applications of these new steroid preparations. The use of these drugs has to be continued until the disease process is completely suppressed. Topical steroids should be used in short courses, and not indefinitely once the lesion has resolved. If there is relapse then the steroid should be used again.

*Systemic steroids.* In patients with plaques resistant to topical corticosteroids, systemic steroids at a dose of prednisone 30 mg per day are usually effective within a few weeks. A maintenance dose of approximately 10 mg per day is sometimes necessary until the disease burns itself out.

**Figure 17.5** *Scarring due to long-standing discoid lupus erythematosus.*

**Figure 17.6** *Discoid lupus erythematosus, with involvement of the lip, presenting as a persistent ulcer.*

**Figure 17.7** *Typical patch of discoid lupus erythematosus on the cheek and a bald area on the scalp caused by the same disorder.*

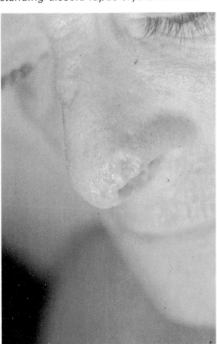

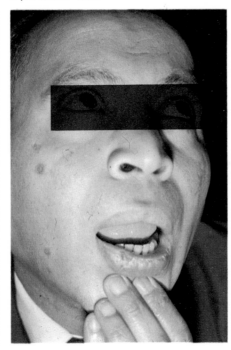

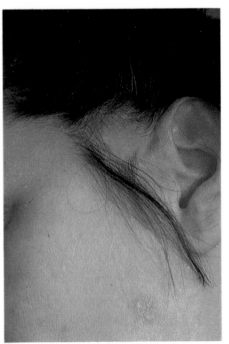

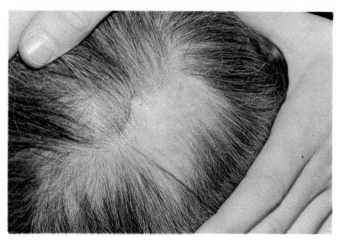

**Figure 17.8** *Hair loss due to discoid lupus erythematosus. There is atrophy of the skin which is still red and scaly.*

*Anti-malarial drugs.* Chloroquine is often effective in controlling the skin lesions, but its use is probably not justified any longer, because of the risk of damage to retina and cornea, even after short courses of the drug.

### Systemic Lupus Erythematosus

As the name implies this is a systemic disorder which may or may not have cutaneous manifestations. It is essentially a vasculitis and organs may be involved either singly or together.

The presenting symptoms of systemic LE are numerous, but the commoner ones are skin lesions, PUO, fatigue,

arthropathy, renal involvement and pleural or pericardial effusions.

Approximately half the patients with systemic LE have skin lesions. Although the cutaneous manifestations are not constant or regular, they may in some cases present with clinical patterns which are distinct enough to suggest the diagnosis. The face is the commonest site to be involved and the 'classical' eruption is the 'butterfly' outline on the nose and malar prominences (Figure 17.9). At first this is simply an erythema but with more severe involvement the erythema increases and approaches the appearances of a cellulitis even showing exudation and crusting. Frequently the eruption will be more extensive, all the exposed areas being involved with diffuse erythema, and it may finally become generalised involving the unexposed areas (Figure 17.10). Hair loss of a diffuse type occurs in a small percentage of patients and has been known to be the presenting symptom. The skin lesions when they resolve do not scar as with the chronic discoid type of LE but they often leave residual hyperpigmentation.

There are often telangiectasia on the posterior nail folds and splinter haemorrhages on the nail bed. The knees and elbows may show erythema, telangiectasia, and scaling which occasionally breaks down and ulcerates. Occasionally these lesions may be seen at other parts of the body. Very rarely the presenting sign is purpura due to thrombocytopenia.

### Diagnosis

Skin biopsy for routine histological study may show only non-specific inflammatory changes. Direct immunofluores-

**Figure 17.9** *Systemic lupus erythematosus presenting as confluent erythema on the nose and cheeks. There is also involvement of the chin and upper lip.*

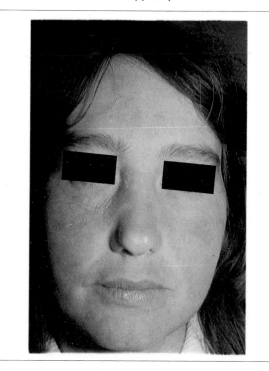

**Figure 17.10** *Systemic lupus erythematosus. Eruption becoming generalised and involving non-exposed as well as exposed areas. The eruption on the upper arm is symmetrical and there is some scaling which occurs in the more acute forms of the disease.*

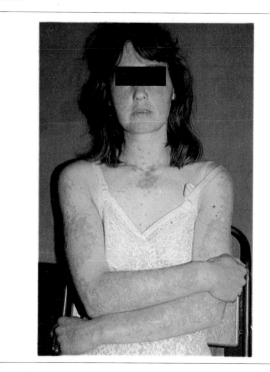

cent studies show deposition of IgG in the region of the basement membrane. This finding is *also* present in the exposed and uninvolved skin. The band of IgG is much wider and more irregular than that found in pemphigoid.

Serological studies show the presence of antinuclear antibodies. These are present in all patients, but they may not appear for some time after the clinical onset of symptoms. LE cells are present in approximately half the patients, but it should be remembered that they are not specific for systemic lupus erythematosus.

### Treatment and Prognosis

The management of systemic lupus erythematosus will vary according to the clinical extent of the disease, which organs are involved, and the severity of involvement. Systemic steroids are still the most useful drugs in the acute stages of the disease, although immunosuppressive drugs such as azathioprine are being used more frequently, particularly when the disease enters a more chronic phase. Not infrequently the disease will go into remission, and then the dose of steroids and immunosuppressive drugs can be reduced and in some cases stopped.

Although the cause of systemic lupus erythematosus is unknown, sunlight is best avoided as it can produce an acute exacerbation in some patients. Some drugs such as penicillin and procaine amide have been known to produce a lupus erythematosus-like illness completely reversible when the drug is stopped and this induced type usually has an excellent prognosis. The prognosis of 'non drug induced' systemic lupus erythematosus is variable. It may prove fatal within a short space of time, while in others the disease will smoulder on and produce death usually due to renal involvement. However, the disease is not invariably fatal although the morbidity is high. In some instances there may be acute exacerbations from time to time with general good health in between.

## Scleroderma

As with LE there are two types of scleroderma, a 'localised cutaneous' form and a systemic form which has cutaneous manifestations.

### Localised Scleroderma

This is sometimes referred to as 'morphoea'. It consists of hardened plaques in the dermis with overlying atrophic epidermis. The lesions may occur at any site, they are usually round or oval but may be linear. In the early stages the lesion presents as a firm white plaque (Figures 17.11 and 17.12) often with a surrounding violaceous hue, which subsequently becomes pigmented (Figure 17.12). If the area is particularly hairy, loss of hair will be noted. If the face is involved there may be underlying atrophy of the muscles. There is usually no systemic involvement associated with morphoea.

### Prognosis and Treatment

In the majority of patients the lesions will tend to improve gradually and there may be complete resolution although this may not occur for five to ten years. The cause is unknown

**Figure 17.11** *Localised scleroderma (morphoea) on the back of the hand.*

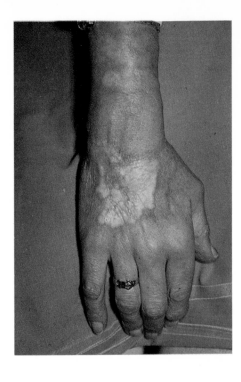

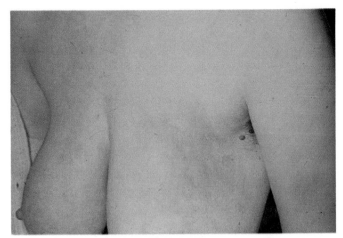

**Figure 17.12** *White area of morphoea with surrounding area of pigmentation.*

**Figure 17.13** *The systemic form of scleroderma. The skin becomes tight, leading to immobility and deformity of the hands.*

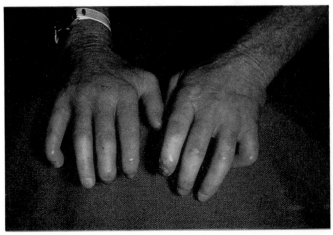

and unfortunately there is no effective treatment at the present time.

### Systemic Scleroderma

This is a chronic disorder, sometimes referred to as systemic sclerosis, in which a few or many organs may be involved. The pathological changes are most pronounced in the connective tissue due to alteration of the collagen. The skin is usually involved in the disease and the other systems commonly involved are the gastrointestinal tract and lungs. When the gastrointestinal tract is affected there is usually involvement of the oesophagus with altered peristalsis and ultimately dysphagia. The small intestine may be affected, giving rise to malabsorption, and the large bowel, giving rise to constipation. When the lungs are involved there is a diffusion defect. The kidneys and heart may also be affected.

The skin changes are often preceded by Raynaud's phenomenon which may be present for a number of years before the actual skin lesions are apparent. The face, hands and forearms are the commonest sites to be affected. The patient may first notice difficulty in moving the fingers; the skin, which has a shiny appearance, becomes immobile and tight and this may lead to deformity of the hand (Figure 17.13). There may be atrophy of the pulp space on the tips of the fingers giving the appearance of thin, tapering digits (Figures 17.14 and 17.15). The expression on the face may be altered because of tightness of the skin, patients are unable to smile, and may notice they are unable to open their mouths wide enough to put a spoon inside. In the later stages there may be macular patches of telangiectasia on the cheeks. As in systemic lupus erythematosus there may be dilated capillaries and nail fold haemorrhages. Cutaneous calcinosis is a fairly frequent manifestation of systemic sclerosis. It is common on the hands, particularly the tips of the fingers where it may present as persistent ulcers, while elsewhere it presents as hard, white nodules.

#### Prognosis and Treatment

There is a variable prognosis in this disorder. Some patients may die from the disease within a year or two of the first signs appearing, particularly if the heart or kidneys are involved. On the other hand patients may show very slow progression of the disorder over twenty to thirty years and may well die of an intercurrent illness.

Treatment is unsatisfactory. At the present time there is no known measure which can significantly alter the course of the illness. Systemic steroids, other hormones and immunosuppressive agents have all been tried without obvious benefit. Simple measures, such as avoidance of cold if Raynaud's phenomenon is present, and physiotherapy to improve the immobility of the hands and arms are points worth paying attention to.

### Dermatomyositis

Dermatomyositis is a disorder involving skin and skeletal

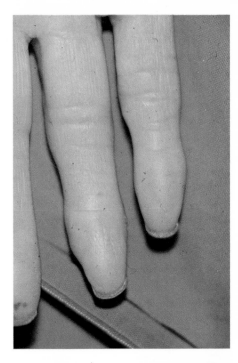

**Figure 17.14**
*Loss of pulp space in the fingers in systemic sclerosis.*

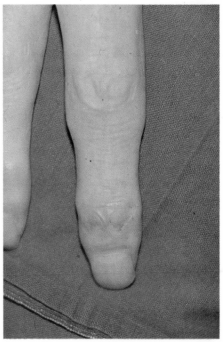

*Figure **17.15** Tapering of the finger, with tight shiny skin in systemic sclerosis.*

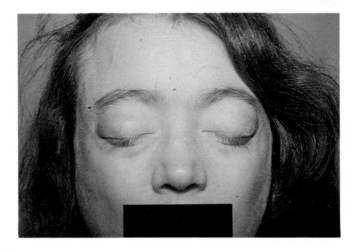

**Figure 17.16** (Right) *Purplish erythema around the eyes in dermatomyositis.*

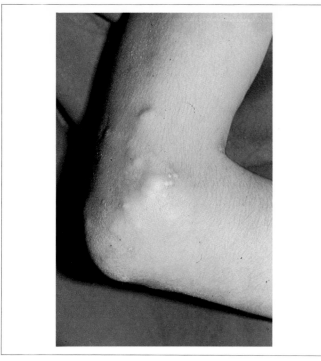

**Figure 17.17** *Cutaneous calcinosis in dermatomyositis around the elbow joint.*

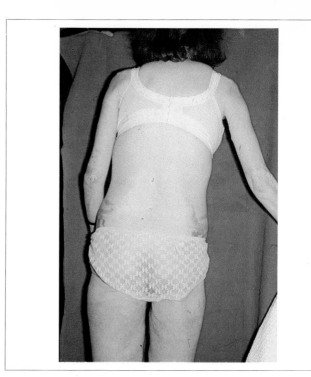

**Figure 17.18** *Wasting of the muscles around shoulders, upper arms, pelvis and thighs in chronic dermatomyositis.*

muscle. It may first present in childhood or adult life. In adults, but not children, the disease is associated with internal malignancy in approximately 50 per cent of cases.

### Skin Lesions

These usually begin around the eyes as a purplish erythema (Figure 17.16). There may be accompanying oedema which in some instances may be so severe as to close the eyes. The neck, chest, arms and occasionally the whole body may be similarly involved. Subsequently the skin may become scaly and occasionally in the severe forms blisters may appear. In the later stages, when the oedema has subsided there is left a reticulate erythema and patchy pigmentation which may progress to atrophic changes in the skin.

As in scleroderma the patients may have Raynaud's phenomenon and develop cutaneous calcinosis. However, in dermatomyositis the calcinosis tends to occur around the joints, particularly the knees and elbows (Figure 17.17). Calcinosis is more likely to occur in the juvenile cases.

### Muscle

*Muscular involvement.* The muscular involvement is variable like the skin lesions. In the mild forms there is weakness of the muscles, usually those of the shoulders, upper arms, pelvic girdle and thighs. The weakness may be minimal and hardly be noticed, but in those more severely involved there will be obvious impairment of muscular activity (e.g. patients often notice the muscle involvement because of difficulty with climbing or descending stairs). In the most severe cases there may be involvement of all muscles, and therefore difficulty with swallowing and breathing, and it is involvement of these muscles which may kill. In the juvenile form the disease tends to be chronic, and severe wasting of the muscles, particularly those of the shoulders (Figure 17.18) and pelvis, occurs.

Occasionally the skin lesions may be severe but the muscle involvement minimal and vice versa.

The diagnosis is usually confirmed by muscle enzyme and electromyographic studies.

### Prognosis and Treatment

The prognosis is variable. Obviously in adults a search must be made for internal malignancy. If the disease is not associated with a carcinoma, dermatomyositis may be fatal itself. In other instances the disease will run a protracted course of many years before burning itself out leaving permanent wasting of muscles. Finally in other patients it may be transient and leave very little residual change in skin or muscle.

In the acute stages large doses of systemic corticosteroids will be needed. Once over the acute stage the dose can be reduced to a maintenance level to stop further muscle damage.

# 18. Naevi and Benign Skin Tumours

NAEVUS is the Latin word for mole and literally means 'blemish' or 'lump' on the skin. There is a certain amount of confusion over its use. Some people use it to imply congenital lesions, i.e. lesions present at birth, but not all naevi are present at birth; and other people use the term to imply benign pigmented lesions. It is probably best used in its literal sense as described above and only with an appropriate adjective to describe the lesion.

## Pigmented Naevi

These are lesions in which melanocytes of the epidermis undergo changes which give rise to specific cells termed 'naevus' cells. The naevus cells may be found wholly in either the epidermis or dermis or in both. Thus, although these cells are derived from the epidermis, they appear to migrate into the dermis. By implication a naevus is a defect in the development of the skin. Not all the melanocytes in a lesion show complete progression to naevus cells. Melanocytes showing only slight changes are often referred to as immature naevus cells whilst those in which the changes are complete are known as mature naevus cells. When there is focal proliferation of melanocytes in the epidermis only (this occurs in the basal layer of the epidermis where melanocytes are found) the naevus is called a 'junctional' naevus, because histologically the change is at the junction of dermis and epidermis. This so-called junctional activity is seen when naevi undergo malignant change, but junctional activity in a naevus does *not* itself imply malignant change. Naevi in which naevus cells are found in the epidermis and dermis are referred to as compound naevi, whilst those in which the cells are wholly dermal are termed intra-dermal naevi. It has been assumed in the past that those naevi which are wholly intra-dermal are unlikely to undergo malignant change. However, this is an assumption which has been challenged. It is argued that even intra-dermal naevi may have some epidermal component which is not seen on a two dimensional microscopical view. However, the implication is that it is only the 'naevus' cells in the epidermis which undergo malignant change.

Pigmented naevi are not all present at birth and may appear in infancy and childhood. They appear to be hormone dependent in some instances, appearing for the first time at puberty, during pregnancy and in persons taking the contraceptive pill.

Every adult has a few pigmented naevi, the number varying greatly. The average is somewhere between 15 and 20. The clinical importance of pigmented naevi (apart from their cosmetic significance) is whether they may develop into malignant melanomata. Everybody has a number of these lesions and malignancy is uncommon, so the chances of malignancy developing are very small indeed.

### Clinical Features

Pigmented naevi can be divided into groups on morphological grounds.

#### Flat Lesions

These are macular pigmented lesions varying in size from a few millimetres to a few centimtres (Figure 18.1). On occasions they may be very extensive and cover very large areas of skin, e.g. half a limb. Histologically, these are 'junctional'. The commonest site is the palms and soles. There is no reason to remove these lesions unless they change their clinical features.

#### Slightly Raised Lesions

Again these vary in size but they are commonly a few millimetres in diameter. Coarse hairs are frequently present. Histologically, they are often referred to as 'compound' as it is easy to see both intradermal and junctional areas on microscopy.

#### Sessile and Dome-shaped Lesions (Figure 18.2)

These frequently bear coarse hairs and histologically are predominantly intradermal. Pigmented naevi, usually the compound or intra-dermal varieties, may be numerous in some persons (Figure 18.3), and there may well be over a hundred on the skin.

**Figure 18.1** *Macular pigmented naevus.*

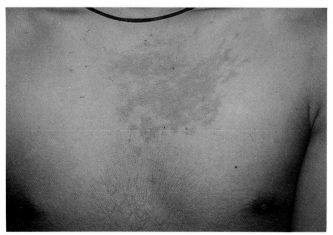

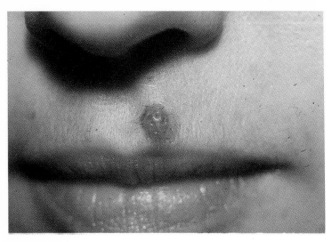

**Figure 18.2** *The common pigmented naevus. The lesion is raised and often dome-shaped, and coarse hairs are frequently present.*

**Figure 18.3** *Numerous pigmented naevi. There is variation in size and elevation of the lesions.*

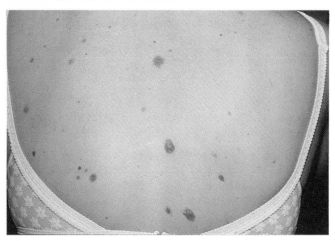

**Figure 18.4**
*Epidermal or warty naevus. The lesions are often linear.*

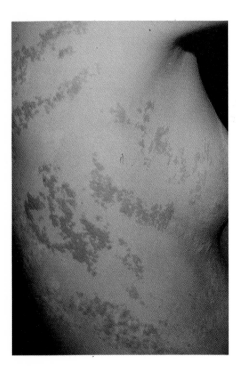

### Epidermal or Warty Naevi

Histologically these lesions are different from the pigmented naevi described above. They do not appear to arise from melanocytes, but consist of a proliferation of the epidermal cells (keratinocytes). However, there is often increased melanocytic activity. Clinically the lesions present as raised, warty (rough surface with clefts) lesions and are often linear. These lesions may be extensive (Figure 18.4).

### Treatment and Management

There are three main reasons for removing pigmented naevi. First, and most important, they should be removed if it is suspected that they are becoming malignant. A lesion should be suspected of malignancy if:

1. It suddenly enlarges.

2. There is an alteration in the pigmentation of the lesion itself or of the surrounding skin.

3. If there is bleeding or ulceration of the lesion.

The second reason for removal is if the lesion is prominent and situated on part of the skin which is subjected to trauma from clothing, e.g. brassiere straps, and is causing discomfort to the part. The third, and probably the commonest, reason for removal is cosmetic.

All pigmented naevi that are to be removed should be surgically excised whatever the indication. No other forms of therapy should be attempted.

### Juvenile Melanoma

This is a term applied to a naevus which usually appears in childhood and grows rapidly. On microscopy the features are similar to those seen in a malignant melanoma but a juvenile melanoma is always benign. As a general rule pigmented naevi do not undergo malignant change prior to puberty.

### Basal Cell Papilloma or Seborrhoeic Wart

These lesions are very common. They are not caused by viruses. Seborrhoeic warts are disorders of middle aged and elderly persons. They are usually oval or circular and most frequently occur on the face and trunk. Initially they grow fairly rapidly and then remain stationary. The lesions are pigmented, have a cleft surface and greasy appearance, hence the name seborrhoeic (Figures 18.5 and 18.6). They do not regress like viral warts and they do not become malignant. If the patient wants them removed, the procedure should be curettage and cautery under local anaesthetic.

### Skin Tags or Fibro-epithelial Polyps

These usually occur in middle aged persons. The commonest sites are the neck and axillae (Figure 18.7). They may be few or many in number. They are benign and are easily removed by snipping the base with scissors and then cauterising to stop bleeding.

### Histiocytoma

This is a fairly common tumour. It is found more frequently in females than males and the commonest site is the legs

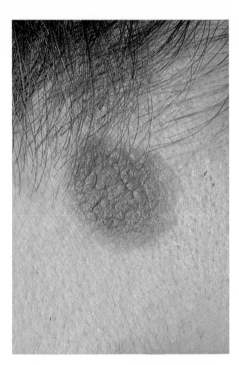

**Figure 18.5**
*Typical seborrhoeic wart. The lesion is pigmented, raised, and has a cleft surface and a greasy appearance.*

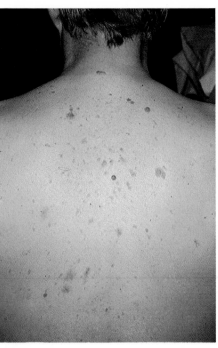

**Figure 18.6**
*Numerous seborrhoeic warts on the trunk. The lesions are often multiple.*

**Figure 18.7**
(Below)
*Skin tags or fibroepithelial polyps. The commonest sites are the neck and axillae.*

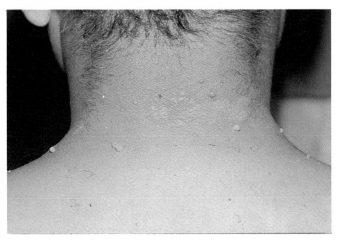

below the knees. These lesions are in the dermis and therefore the surface is smooth as the overlying epidermis is not affected. They present as firm nodules varying from approximately 0.5 to 2.0 centimetres in diameter. The cause of histiocytomata is unknown but it has been postulated that they follow trauma. The lesions are benign and not infrequently are numerous. The only treatment available is surgical excision.

### Keloids

These are formed by an abnormal response to trauma by the connective tissue of the dermis. Excess collagen is formed. Undoubtedly the commonest cause of a keloid is surgery (Figure 18.8), but the lesions are also seen following trauma and infection of the dermis whether viral or bacterial. In Asians and negroes spontaneous keloids occur usually on the trunk (Figure 18.9) and upper arms. Keloids are commoner in negroes than in caucasians and this should be borne in mind before embarking on removal of benign skin tumours in negroes. Clinically a keloid is a raised, firm lesion with a smooth surface (normal epidermis). If it presents at the site of surgery or trauma, there is no difficulty in diagnosis (Figure 18.8), but spontaneous keloids may present diagnostic problems (Figure 18.9). The treatment of keloids has improved recently, with the advent of intralesional steroid therapy. Intralesional injections of triamcinolone will result in the shrinkage of the keloid due to the action of the steroid on collagen. The treatment should be carried out early, as 'young collagen' responds more readily to the action of the steroid. Keloids should not be excised; if a patient has a tendency to form keloids, another keloid will almost certainly occur following surgery for the original lesion.

### Haemangiomata

These may be divided into congenital and acquired types. The former may be further subdivided into those arising from immature vessels and those arising from mature vessels.

### Immature Haemangiomata (Strawberry Naevi)

These are only very rarely present at birth. They usually appear within the first week of life as a small red spot and then rapidly enlarge. They are raised above the skin surface and deep red in colour (Figure 18.10). These haemangiomata may continue to enlarge until the age of eighteen months though frequently they stop increasing in size before then. The eventual size they attain varies considerably; they may simply be a few millimetres in diameter or as large as 10 centimetres in diameter. After eighteen months size and appearance usually do not change but after the age of 3 years they begin to shrink and become paler (Figure 18.11) and should disappear completely by the age of 5 or 6 years.

### Management and Treatment

From the natural history it can be seen that all lesions will disappear. If there is any residual scarring or puckering of the skin this can be dealt with after complete resolution. The best cosmetic result will be obtained if the lesions are not

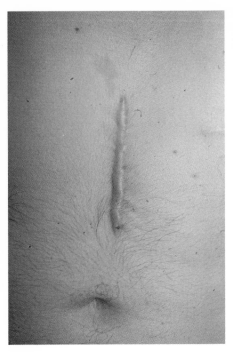

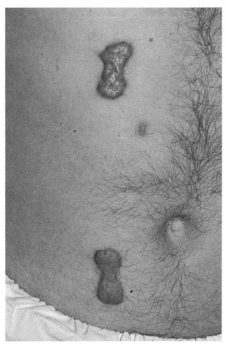

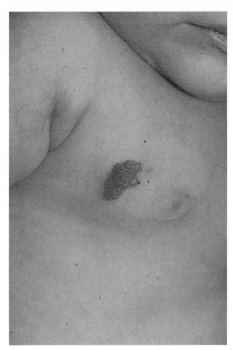

**Figure 18.8** *Keloid developing in a surgical scar.*

**Figure 18.9** *Spontaneous keloids. Firm, nodular plaques on the trunk.*

**Figure 18.10** *Immature capillary haemangioma (strawberry naevus).*

treated at all. Occasionally, if the haemangioma is near the eye its growth could 'close' the eye and hence interfere with the development of binocular vision. In these instances the lesion can be made to resolve by radiotherapy.

### Mature Haemangiomata (Port-wine Stain)

These lesions are present in full extent at birth which distinguishes them from the immature haemangiomata. They are macular (Figure 18.12). Unfortunately, they persist throughout life and do not undergo any resolution. These haemangiomata may vary from a few centimetres to many in size. The commonest site is the neck. They are a severe cosmetic disability, particularly if extensive.

The only treatment at present is to cover them by a suitable covering cream and many cosmetic firms now prepare such creams which can be made to blend in with the natural colour of the patient's skin. The lesions are not sensitive to X-irradiation.

### Deep Haemangiomata

A small percentage of mature haemangiomata are raised and are related to abnormalities of the deeper vessels.

### Acquired Haemangiomata

1. *Pyogenic granuloma.* This lesion is so-called because it was thought to be due to infection by a staphylococcus. It is usually a solitary raised papule, red in colour (Figure 18.13) and bleeds on the slightest trauma. It may occur anywhere on the body. The cause is unknown but sometimes there is a history of preceding trauma. The most effective treatment is curettage and cautery under local anaesthetic.

**Figure 18.11** *Immature capillary naevus beginning to resolve. The centre of the lesion becomes paler, and the lesion begins to flatten.*

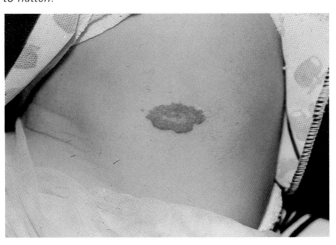

2. *Campbell de Morgan spots* (*cherry angiomata*). These are small raised bright red angiomata (Figure 18.14) which tend to occur on the trunk in middle-aged and elderly persons. They are relatively common but they have no special clinical significance. No treatment is indicated but they can be removed by surgery or cautery.

3. '*Spider naevi*'. These are common lesions occurring at any age. There is a small central red papule from which superficial vessels radiate (Figure 18.15). They usually occur on the face, arms, hands and upper trunk. The lesions are usually solitary and do not imply any internal disease. However, occasionally they are multiple and are due to

114

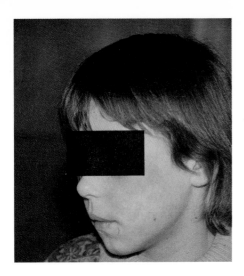

**Figure 18.12**
*Mature capillary haemangioma (port-wine stain). The lesion is usually macular and persists.*

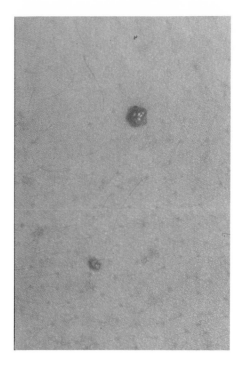

**Figure 18.14**
*Campbell de Morgan spots (acquired haemangiomata). The commonest site is on the trunk.*

**Figure 18.13** *Pyogenic granuloma (acquired haemangioma).*

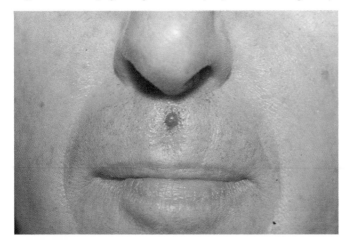

**Figure 18.15** *Spider naevus. A central red 'dot' with small vessels radiating away from the centre.*

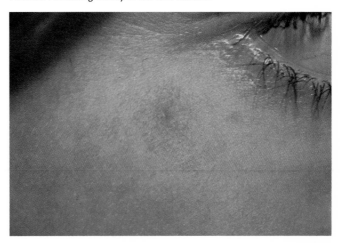

underlying liver disease. They may also appear in pregnancy, frequently disappearing after the confinement.

If treatment is required, the most satisfactory is cautery to the central papule without local anaesthetic. If the latter is used it causes vasoconstriction and the central papule is no longer visible.

### Hereditary Telangiectasia

This is a rare but important disease. Small haemangiomata are present on the face, lips and tongue. The importance of the disease lies in the fact that the haemangiomata also occur in the gastrointestinal tract and may bleed causing a severe haemorrhage. If there is a large bleed, the fall in blood pressure results in the 'disappearance' of the haemangiomata on the face and lips and so the diagnosis is missed.

### Lymphangiomata

This is a relatively rare lesion. It presents as grouped blisters on any part of the body. The blisters are deep and the fluid can be easily 'pressed out'. Frequently there are haemangiomatous elements associated with a lymphangioma so the lesion may have a vascular appearance. The only treatment available is surgery but unfortunately there is a high recurrence rate.

# 19. Urticaria and Erythema Multiforme

URTICARIA is sometimes referred to as 'hives' or 'nettle rash' by patients. Urticaria is basically localised oedema of the skin or mucous membranes of the upper respiratory tract. It is caused by acute vasodilatation of the blood vessels and increased permeability of the capillary walls with fluid pouring out into the dermis with resultant swelling of the skin. The vasodilatation and increased permeability is caused by various chemical mediators in the skin which are released under certain conditions. Histamine is one of the substances which can cause an urticarial response and this can be shown quite simply by the injection of histamine into the skin.

However, it is now thought that in urticaria histamine is only one of many substances which cause the clinical lesion.

## Morphology

The initial lesion is an erythematous patch (there is no scaling in urticaria) caused by capillary vasodilatation. The lesion subsequently becomes raised (Figures 19.1, 19.2 and 19.3) and may finally have a white centre caused by the pressure of intercellular fluid forcing the blood out of the capillaries (Figures 19.3, 19.4 and 19.5). The actual size of an urticarial lesion may vary from a few mm to many cm (Figure 19.1) and, on occasions involves large confluent areas of skin (Figures 19.2, 19.4 and 19.6). The urticarial lesions often have a 'geographic' pattern, rather than any regular configuration. If the palms or soles are involved, the typical urticarial pattern is not present, the affected area being tense, red and swollen. When the fingers or toes are affected the swelling may interfere with movement. Urticaria not infrequently involves the face, when an alarming picture is produced with swelling around the eyes (Figure 19.7) and/or lips so that gross disfiguration is produced. When urticaria takes this pattern it is sometimes referred to as angioneurotic oedema (not a particularly good term).

Urticarial skin lesions may be associated with swelling of the tongue, pharynx and larynx. This is a serious happening as the patient may asphyxiate. The condition may occur within minutes of the first symptoms appearing.

Organs other than the skin may be affected in association with urticaria (whatever the cause of the latter), e.g. swelling of the joints, bronchospasm, the gut (in the form of colicky abdominal pains), and very rarely there is anaphylactic shock.

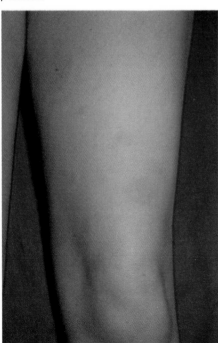

**Figure 19.1** *Mild urticaria. Raised, red patches.*

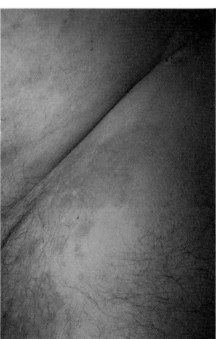

**Figure 19.2** *Raised, red plaques of urticaria.*

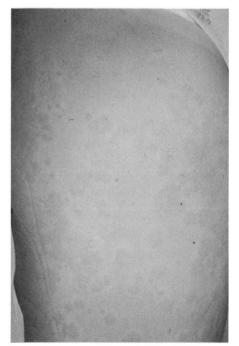

**19.3** *Raised red patches, some with white centres, in urticaria.*

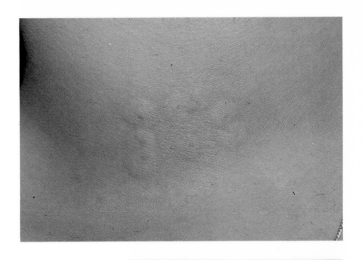

## Course

An actual urticarial lesion tends to last for a few hours, although it may last for as little as a few minutes and, occasionally, for as long as a few days. When the lesion first forms it is intensely irritating. In patients who give a long history of urticaria, it is important to establish that an individual lesion does, in fact, 'come and go'. In those patients who are never free from the eruption it is not the original lesions which persist. Lesions as stated above tend to last for a few hours and then clear but new lesions will appear at other sites.

The natural history of urticaria is variable. It depends to a certain extent upon whether there are any obvious precipitating factors. In the patients in whom there are no obvious precipitating factors the disease may last from a few days to many years. In some instances the patient is never free of lesions, in others they may be clear for a few days or even weeks but the rash then recurs. Urticaria may also run a variable course in those patients in whom there is an obvious cause (e.g. penicillin). It may last for only a few days or may persist for weeks despite no further penicillin intake.

## Causes

In the majority of patients with chronic urticaria seen in a skin clinic no cause is found for the eruption. In an acute episode, which is often self-limiting, it is much more common to find a cause.

### Drugs

These are the most common known cause of urticaria seen today. Penicillin is the most frequent offender but com-

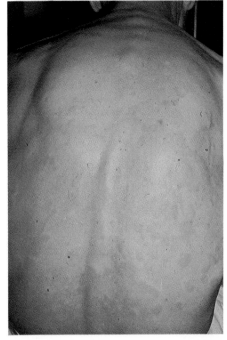

**Figure 19.6**
*Bizarre configuration of the lesions often seen in extensive urticaria.*

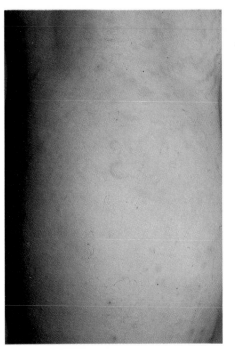

**Figure 19.4**
*Raised, irregular plaque in urticaria. The lesion is becoming paler as the disorder becomes more severe.*

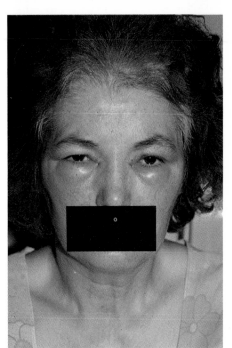

**Figure 19.7**
*Swelling around the eyes in angioneurotic oedema.*

117

pounds containing salicylates also produce a relatively high incidence of urticarial eruptions. As mentioned in the chapter on 'Drug Eruptions' any drug can cause any rash, so it is important to ask patients who have urticaria if they have taken (or been given) any drugs in the last few months. The number of drugs known to produce urticaria is now so numerous that it would be of no help to name them here, but, apart from drugs taken orally or given by injection, it is important to remember that inhaled medication or drugs absorbed through a mucous membrane have also to be considered when searching for the offending substance. It is also important to find out whether the patient has received any inoculations or blood transfusions.

### Foods

In most cases of urticaria the patient assumes that some particular food is the cause. Certainly in chronic urticaria this is very rarely the case. Usually, if a patient is sensitive to a particular food there is a definite history of ingestion of this food just before the eruption. The most common food to cause urticaria is probably shell-fish. I think it unwise to specify other foods but ask the patient whether any particular food was ingested before the rash appeared. Elimination diets and skin testing have not proved of any help in establishing whether the patient is sensitive to a particular food. However, these procedures often have a 'negative' therapeutic value for when carried out and shown to be negative, they help to convince the patient that he is not ingesting the causative agent of his skin trouble.

Apart from the food itself, certain food additives have been implicated as the cause of chronic urticaria. Tartrazine and other azo dyes are used as colouring substances in food and it has been claimed that they cause urticaria. It should also be mentioned that the same dyes are often used to colour tablets (including antihistamines given in the treatment of urticaria). Preservatives such as sodium benzoate and benzoic acid have also been mentioned as possible aetiological factors. The foods which contain such preservatives are pickles, sauces, instant coffee, preserves, fruit juices and some tinned food.

It has been suggested that challenge doses of these dyes and preservatives should be given, by mouth, to determine whether they are the cause of urticaria, and if there is considered to be a positive response (worsening or induction of urticaria) then a diet free of these substances should be taken. It should be stressed that this approach to the problem is an oversimplification, for in practice it is difficult to evaluate the provocation test, and even if positive results are obtained, elimination does *not* result in a 100 per cent cure.

## Physical Factors

### Heat

In some subjects heat, from whatever source, will produce urticarial lesions. The lesions usually appear within minutes or a few hours of the increase in temperature of the skin. In a number of patients exercise will produce urticaria. This form of urticaria may have the morphology of the lesions

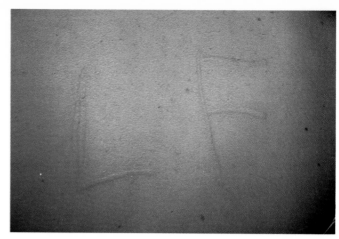

**Figure 19.8** *Dermographism, urticaria in the lines of trauma.*

described above or consist of very small (2–3 mm) but numerous weals. It is thought that the chemical mediator may be acetylcholine, and this type of urticaria has been termed cholinergic.

### Cold

Cold may also produce urticaria. It usually occurs on the exposed areas of the arms or legs. Two types of cold urticaria have been described; that which occurs within minutes of the skin temperature falling and that which may appear many hours later. The history of cold urticaria can be substantiated by applying a block of ice to the skin for a few minutes and then observing the response.

### Trauma

In some individuals trauma to the skin produces urticarial lesions. These may appear within two to three minutes or, like 'cold urticaria', develop several hours later. This type of urticarial response has been termed 'dermographism'. It can easily be substantiated by stroking the skin with a blunt instrument and the urticaria follows in the line of trauma (Figure 19.8).

### Sunlight

Some persons develop urticaria on areas exposed to the rays of the sun. This is referred to as solar urticaria and is caused by release of chemicals in the skin caused by ultra-violet irradiation.

### Psychogenic Factors

There is no doubt that urticaria is aggravated by tension, worry, stress, etc. but so are many other diseases. It cannot be stated with any certainty whether or not urticaria is actually caused by these factors.

### Internal Diseases

There are recorded instances of urticaria in association with carcinomata, reticulosis, hepatic disorders, renal disorders and collagen diseases. However, whether the underlying systemic disease is directly causing the urticaria, or is coincidental, has yet to be determined.

## Treatment and Management

An accurate history is important in the management of urticaria. It is imperative to know whether any drugs had been taken before the eruption and if they can be implicated. If they can, then they must be avoided in the future. If the patient is still taking drugs they should be stopped or substituted, if possible. There is, today, no reliable test in vitro or in vivo for finding out whether a particular drug is the cause of the eruption. If the eruption is of sudden onset then it may be worth enquiring about any particular food, such as shell-fish, which the patient does not usually take. As mentioned above, skin tests to try and determine the cause of urticaria have not proved helpful. Oral provocation tests with drugs and food additives may be tried, but as already noted they are difficult to evaluate, as are the results of elimination diets, in a disease with such a variable course. If it can be established that urticaria is caused by physical factors, then the appropriate advice should be given to minimise the effects of these factors.

### Antihistamines

These drugs are the mainstay in the treatment of urticaria. They are usually given orally, but in severe and acute urticaria they can be given by intramuscular or intravenous injection to obtain quicker control of the condition. Which antihistamine to use is usually the personal choice of the doctor. All antihistamines appear to have a similar therapeutic effect, but some tend to cause drowsiness (the main side-effect of these drugs) more readily than others. At night, however, it may be helpful to have a drug which has the effect of making patients drowsy and trimeprazine tartrate or promethazine hydrochloride would appear to be the best drugs for this purpose. A number of antihistamines are now made as 'slow-release' or 'long-acting' tablets and they are sometimes helpful in minimising the soporific effect. Long-acting chlorpheniramine maleate has proved helpful in chronic urticaria. It appears to be possible to give a large dose of antihistamine and obtain a therapeutic effect without making the patient drowsy. Often urticaria is not controlled because the dose of antihistamine given is too small. The dose of antihistamine should be increased until the urticaria is controlled or until side-effects from the antihistamine are intolerable.

### Corticosteroids

These drugs should only be used in emergencies such as angioneurotic oedema with involvement of the tongue and larynx. Corticosteroids are also indicated in anaphylactoid shock. In both instances they should be given intravenously. Systemic corticosteroids should not be used to try to control chronic urticaria. They do not appear to be as effective as antihistamines and on a long-term basis are far more hazardous. Topical corticosteroids have no part to play in the treatment of urticaria.

### Adrenaline

Subcutaneous adrenaline is still one of the most effective

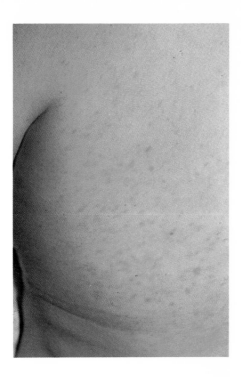

**Figure 19.9** *Numerous brown macules on the trunk in urticaria pigmentosa.*

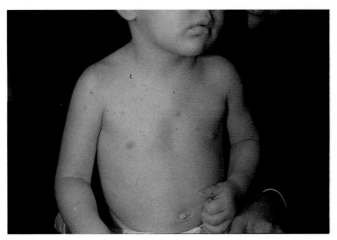

**Figure 19.10** *Urticaria pigmentosa. Pigmented papules on the trunk.*

**Figure 19.11** *Urticaria produced by trauma to the lesion in urticaria pigmentosa. The pigmentation in the centre of the lesion is still visible.*

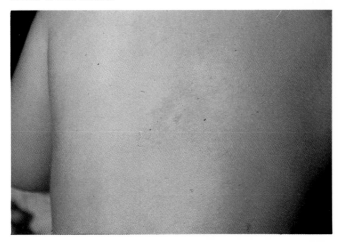

119

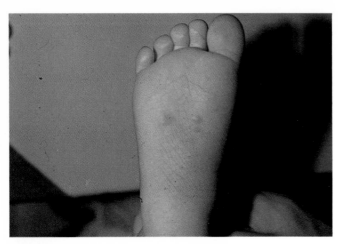

Figure 19.12 *Blisters in urticaria pigmentosa.*

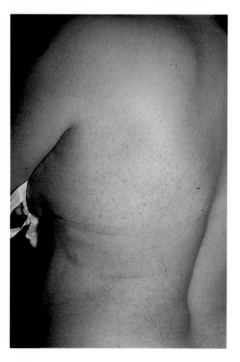

**Figure 19.14**
*Reddish-brown
macules in adult
mastocytosis.*

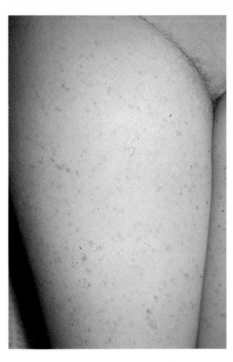

**Figure 19.13**
*Numerous brown
macules on the
trunk in
acquired or adult
mastocytosis.*

**Figure 19.15** *Symmetrical urticarial plaques on the back in
erythema multiforme.*

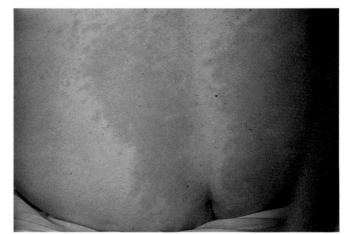

measures in controlling acute urticaria, particularly when
there is involvement of the mouth and larynx.

### Tracheotomy

This would be indicated as an emergency procedure if the
the patient were asphyxiating because of laryngeal and
pharyngeal swelling.

### Topical Measures

Because the epidermis is intact in urticaria, topical drugs
do not penetrate to the site of pathology in therapeutic
concentrations. Topical measures are, therefore, of no use
in urticaria.

### Psychotropic Drugs

Drugs to control anxiety and depression should only be
used if there are specific indications.

## Urticaria Pigmentosa (Mastocytosis)

This is a disorder caused by tumours of mast cells. There are
two distinct forms of urticaria pigmentosa, one which
occurs in childhood and another which appears in later life.

### Childhood Variety

The lesions may be present at birth or appear within the
first few months of life. The most common lesion is a small
pigmented macule occurring predominantly on the trunk
(Figure 19.9). The lesions may be few or very numerous
(Figure 19.9). Occasionally, they present as small pigmented
papules (Figure 19.10) or nodules. The diagnosis is made
by gently scratching the lesions. This slight trauma releases
histamine from the mast cells and an acute urticarial lesion
develops (Figure 19.11). Occasionally there is a more severe
response and blisters occur (Figure 19.12). The parents of
the child will often notice urticarial lesions after slight

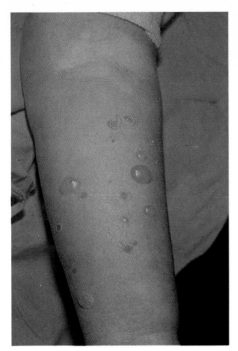

**Figure 19.16** *Urticarial plaque and blisters in erythema multiforme.*

**Figure 19.17** *'Target' lesions in erythema multiforme.*

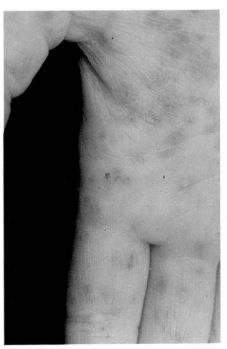

**Figure 19.18** *Erythematous macular lesions with central pupura, an early stage in the development of target lesions.*

trauma to the child's skin such as drying after bathing. The natural history of childhood or congenital mastocytosis is that the lesions usually disappear by adulthood.

### Adult Variety

This is sometimes referred to as 'acquired mastocytosis'. The lesions may appear at any time and are few in number but slowly become more numerous (Figure 19.13). They are similar to the lesions of congenital or childhood masto-cytosis although the lesions may have a redder appearance (Figure 19.14). It is thought that the adult variety is a form of reticulosis and mast cell tumours develop at other sites, notably the liver, spleen and bones. The disease may progress into an acute form of a reticulosis and the patient die of the disease. The course of the disease is over many years, and it may take 20 to 30 years from the development of the skin lesions to the more serious aspects of the disorder.

There is no treatment for mastocytosis. If the disease becomes an acute reticulosis then the appropriate cytotoxic drugs can be given.

### Erythema Multiforme

This is a distinct symptom complex with an appropriate name because the lesions are of varying morphology. The primary pathology of erythema multiforme is that of a vasculitis in the skin.

### Morphology and Distribution of Lesions

In erythema multiforme the lesions may be erythematous macules or papules, urticarial, purpuric or blistering. There may be one (Figure 19.15) or two (Figure 19.16) of the types of lesion described or all the various types may be present in an individual patient. In the classical form of erythema multiforme the initial lesion is an erythematous macule which transforms to a papule (or blister) and this extends peripherally with central clearing (Figure 19.17). As the border extends a new lesion frequently develops in the centre, which may be purpuric (Figure 19.18), and as many as three or four rings may be noted. This gives rise to so-called 'iris' or 'target' lesions.

The most common site for erythema multiforme is the extremities of the upper limbs (Figures 19.19 and 19.20). The eruption in erythema multiforme is symmetrical (Figures 19.15, 19.19 and 19.20). Occasionally, the lesions may be widespread, occurring on the trunk and limbs and producing confluent lesions (Figure 19.15). In a severe form of the disorder known as the 'Stevens-Johnson syndrome' there is involvement of the mucous membranes of the mouth (Figure 19.21), eyes and genitalia (Figure 19.22). Very occasionally the eye lesions become very severe extending to an iritis, uveitis and even panophthalmitis.

### Course

In the mild form of erythema multiforme the lesions are often asymptomatic and clear within two to three weeks of onset. Occasionally, there may be slight constitutional upset with the onset of the lesions. In the more severe forms the patient may be extremely ill with fever and headache. In some patients with the Stevens-Johnson syndrome the disease may prove fatal.

It is not uncommon for patients to develop recurrent attacks of erythema multiforme, the interval between the episodes varying from a few weeks to a few years.

### Aetiology

The exact cause of erythema multiforme is unknown but it

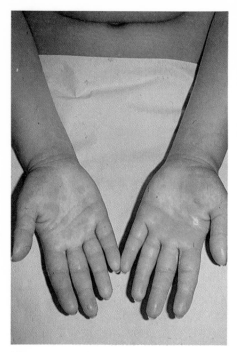

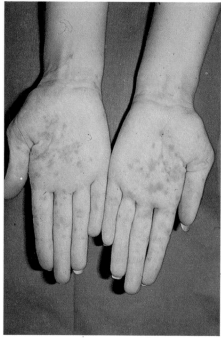

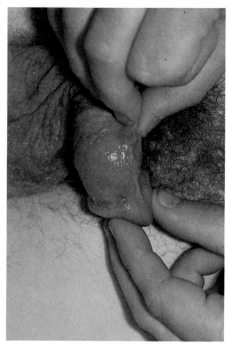

**Figure 19.19** *Symmetrical urticarial lesions on the hands, the commonest site for erythema multiforme.*

**Figure 19.20** *Symmetrical eruption on the hands in erythema multiforme. Macular, vesicular and purpuric lesions are present.*

**Figure 19.22** *Stevens-Johnson syndrome. Ulcers on the genitalia.*

**Figure 19.21** *Stevens-Johnson syndrome. Ulcers on the lips and in the mouth.*

**Figure 19.23** *Erythema multiforme triggered off by herpes simplex infection. The end stage of the herpes simplex infection is present on the lip, and the erythema multiforme has been present for only two days.*

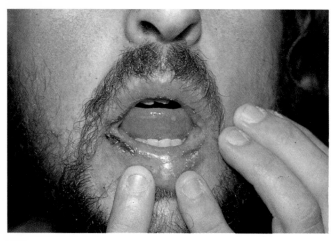

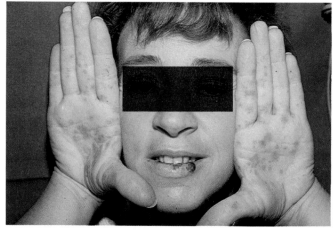

is probably an immunological disorder with the cutaneous blood vessels being the target for the end result of the disease process. In the majority of patients there is no obvious precipitating factor but the following have been recorded as precipitating attacks.

*Viral infections*, particularly herpes simplex (Figure 19.23), but vaccinia and measles have also been found to trigger off the condition.

*Bacterial infections*, particularly streptococcal but also meningococcal infections.

*Mycoplasma*. This organism has been implicated in the causation of erythema multiforme and it is the one which also causes so-called 'primary atypical pneumonia'.

*Drugs*. Particularly sulphonamides and barbiturates, but any drug may cause erythema multiforme.

*Radiotherapy* in the treatment of malignancy has been implicated as precipitating erythema multiforme.

### Treatment and Management

In the mild forms of the disease no treatment is required as the disease is self-limiting. If there is irritation systemic antihistamines should be given. In the more severe forms, particularly the Stevens-Johnson syndrome, systemic corticosteroids are required and hospitalisation is necessary.

In all instances a careful history should be taken to see if there is a possible precipitating factor (e.g. a particular drug) which can be avoided in the future.

# 20. Cutaneous Manifestations of Systemic Disorders

THIS title is not satisfactory or precise but it is difficult to think of a better one. It implies that the skin lesions to be discussed are due to primary pathology in another organ or may be part of a generalised disease affecting many tissues. Strictly speaking it could be argued that the majority of skin lesions (e.g. psoriasis, eczema) are the end result of a generalised process whether the primary fault be immunological, genetic or infective. In this chapter those diseases with the end result of the disease process in organs other than, but in addition to, the skin will be discussed.

## Metabolic Diseases

### Diabetes Mellitus

*Necrobiosis lipoidica*. This is the characteristic skin lesion associated with diabetes mellitus. Approximately half the patients presenting with necrobiosis lipoidica will have glycosuria. The other half are usually considered to be latent diabetics and may develop diabetes later in life. The disorder appears to be more common in women than in men.

The lesions characteristically develop on the anterior aspect of the lower leg (Figure 20.1). The initial lesion is usually an erythematous papule or plaque which gradually extends in an annular fashion. Thus, eventually, the lesion has a raised erythematous edge and in the centre of the lesion (where the disease first began) there is thinning of the epidermis and degeneration of the dermal collagen. The skin in the centre of the lesion has a brownish-yellow colour (Figure 20.2) and the underlying small veins in the dermis are visible. Occasionally, the atrophic epidermis breaks down and ulcerates. The lesions tend to be persistent and unfortunately there is no successful treatment. Control of the diabetes, if present, does not appear to influence the lesions. Topically applied and intralesional injections of corticosteroids have been tried but the results have not been impressive.

*Granuloma annulare*. It is probably incorrect to attribute this disorder to diabetes mellitus but some studies have tried to suggest that the basic pathological process is one similar to that seen in other tissues in the body with diabetes.

**Figure 20.1** *Necrobiosis lipoidica. The characteristic site is the anterior aspect of the lower leg and the lesions have a yellowish brown appearance.*

**Figure 20.2** *Necrobiosis lipoidica. Yellowish brown colour, with thinning (atrophy) of the skin. The underlying veins are easily visible.*

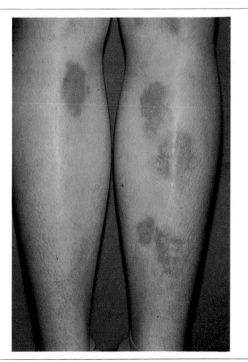

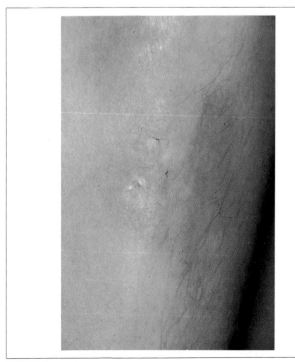

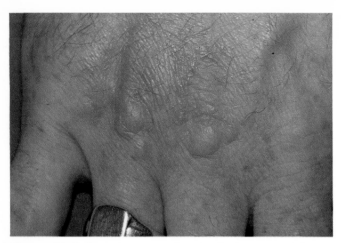

**Figure 20.3** *Granuloma annulare beginning as nodules on the back of the hand.*

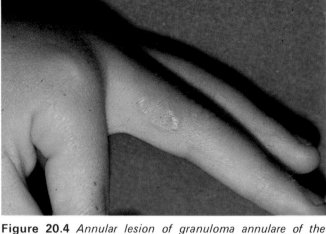

**Figure 20.4** *Annular lesion of granuloma annulare of the finger.*

The lesions characteristically occur on the posterior aspect of the hand (Figure 20.3), fingers (Figure 20.4), extensor surfaces of the elbows and knees and around the ankle joints. They commence as firm papules or nodules (Figure 20.3) in the dermis of the skin. Characteristically, the lesions then extend in an annular pattern with the lesion healing in the centre, thus giving rise to an annular, non-scaling lesion (Figure 20.4). The lesion may be of the normal skin colour or paler but not infrequently it may have a violaceous colour.

The lesions may occur in patients of any age, including young children. As diabetes mellitus appears to be no more common in these patients than in the general population, no particular search for diabetes should be undertaken.

Approximately half the lesions will clear spontaneously within two years of onset. If treatment is required, intra-lesional injections of triamcinolone appear to offer the best chance of cure.

### Xanthomatosis

A xanthoma is a deposit of excess lipids in the skin. Clinically the lesion may appear as a papule, nodule or plaque which has a whitish-yellow colour. The classification may be based on purely clinical morphology, biochemical criteria or in relation to specific underlying disease. There is in any case considerable overlap and here the lesions will be considered under clinical headings. The commonest diseases associated with xanthomata are the primary disorders of lipid metabolism (some of which are hereditary), diabetes mellitus, hypothyroidism, nephrotic syndrome and liver disease (usually biliary cirrhosis).

*Xanthelasma.* This is the commonest form of a xanthoma. It presents as a yellowish-white plaque on the upper eyelid or just below the lower eyelid (Figure 20.5). It usually commences on the medial side of the lid and progresses laterally. It may occur as a single lesion or occur on all four eyelids. Xanthelasmata may occur in subjects who do not have any generalised biochemical disorder but they may be a manifestation of a hyperlipoproteinaemia.

*Nodular xanthomata.* These lesions usually occur on the extensor surfaces of the limbs, particularly over the joint surfaces (Figure 20.6). They present as painless yellowish nodules and vary in size from a few mm to 1–2 cm across.

*Papular xanthomata.* Occasionally, multiple xanthomata appear as numerous small papules over a matter of a few weeks, so called 'eruptive xanthomata'. They usually appear on the trunk or buttocks.

*Plaques.* Lipid deposits in the skin and along the tendon sheaths may present quite often as plaques. They may also be nodular, particularly over large tendons (Figure 20.7).

### Treatment and Management

The treatment of xanthomata will depend on which underlying metabolic disorder has produced the lipid deposits in the skin. Thus, the patient must be investigated to determine whether the lesions are secondary to one of the above mentioned diseases, e.g. diabetes mellitus, or whether they are due to primary hyperlipoproteinaemia. If the lesions

**Figure 20.5** *Xanthelasma. This appears as a yellowish plaque. The skin around the medial aspect of the eyes is the commonest site.*

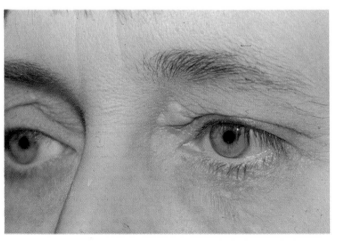

124

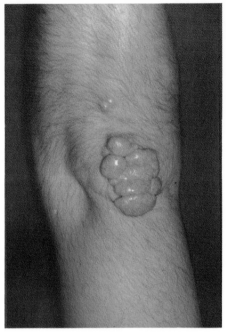

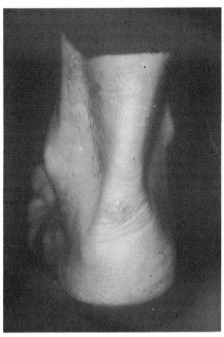

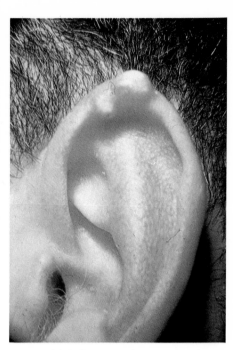

**Figure 20.6** *Nodular xanthomata on the elbow appear as yellowish red nodules.*

**Figure 20.7** *Xanthomata over the Achilles tendon.*

**Figure 20.8** *Gouty tophus on the pinna.*

are secondary then the treatment is that of the primary disorder. If the xanthomata are due to primary hyper-lipoproteinaemia then further investigation is required to determine the biochemical profile, as the treatment by dietary restriction and/or clofibrate will depend on the results.

In patients with xanthelasmata in whom no biochemical disorders are found the lesions may be removed by surgery, or destroyed by electrocautery under local anaesthetic.

### Gout and Rheumatoid Nodules

Gouty tophi usually present as nodules on the ears (Figure 20.8), hands or, occasionally, the extensor surface of the joints of the limbs. The tophus is formed by the deposition of urates in the dermis and subcutis and thus the lesion is frequently attached to the skin. Occasionally the lesion may be present without the classical history of gouty arthritis.

Rheumatoid nodules would not usually present to a dermatologist as the patient would be under the care of a rheumatologist for his 'rheumatic' condition. Occasionally, however, rheumatoid nodules develop in patients who have no joint problems. The commonest sites are the hands but the nodules may also occur in the feet and elbows (Figure 20.9). The lesions are painless.

### Erythema Nodosum

This is a distinct clinical entity. It is a reaction in the skin and subcutaneous tissues (the primary site of pathology being the blood vessels) due to various causes, many of which signify internal disease. The lesions in erythema nodosum occur characteristically on the anterior surface of the legs below the knees (Figure 20.10). Very occasionally they may occur on the posterior surface of the legs, the

extensor surface of the arms and very rarely on the back of the neck. Morphologically, the lesions are red, tender nodules attached to the skin. They may vary in size from 1 cm to 10 cm in diameter. Occasionally, the nodules may join to form a confluent plaque (Figure 20.11). The lesions are painful in the initial stages. They may remain red and tender for two to three weeks, after which they become less painful, turn purple and involute. Not all the lesions will appear simultaneously and thus new ones may be appearing while older ones are beginning to resolve. The pathological process in the skin in erythema nodosum is usually self-limiting and the skin lesions should have cleared within a month of onset.

### Aetiology

The commonest known causes of erythema nodosum are

**Figure 20.9** *Rheumatic nodules on the elbow.*

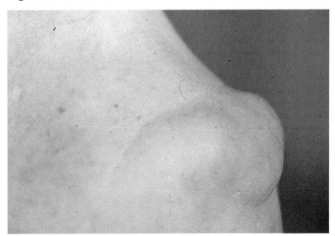

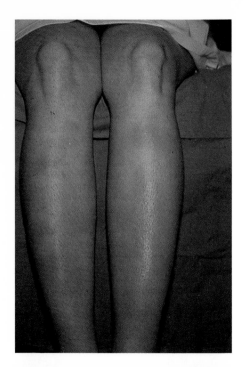

**Figure 20.10**
*Erythema nodosum. The anterior aspect of the leg is a common site for this lesion.*

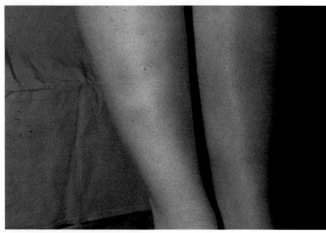

**Figure 20.11**
(Below)
*Confluent plaque forming in erythema nodosum.*

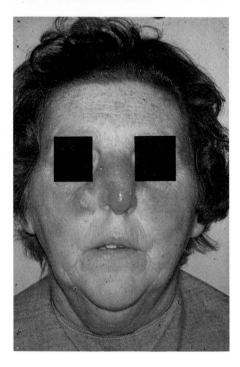

**Figure 20.12**
*Purplish nodules and plaque formation in sarcoidosis of the skin.*

streptococcal infections, primary tuberculous infection, sarcoidosis, and drugs (most frequently sulphonamides—although many other drugs have been recorded as precipitating the condition). Other less frequent causes include meningococcal septicaemia and lymphogranuloma venereum. In some patients no cause is found.

### Management and Treatment

Obviously the most important part of management is to investigate the patient to see whether he is suffering from any of the above mentioned disorders and then, if so, to give the appropriate treatment. The treatment of the actual erythema nodosum lesions will depend on their severity. In the mild forms, rest and simple analgesics are all that is required. In the more severe forms the patient will be more comfortable in bed and if the lesions are very severe, systemic corticosteroids will control the inflammatory response. However, it must be stressed that systemic corticosteroids can only be given *after* the patients have been investigated to try to establish the cause of the condition.

### Sarcoidosis

This is a well recognised clinical entity, with a specific histology, but the aetiology still remains unknown. Sarcoidosis was, in fact, first noted as a skin disorder but has subsequently been found to involve any or all organs. Sarcoidosis in the skin may, therefore, be part of general involvement of the body by the process, or it may be the only organ affected.

The skin lesions are due to dermal or subcutaneous granulomatous infiltrates. They therefore appear as smooth papules, nodules or plaques (Figure 20.12). The lesions may be skin-coloured, pink or purplish. The commonest sites to be affected are the face, neck and hands. A condition in which the skin of the nose, cheeks and ears becomes infiltrated, congested and purplish is now recognised as being a manifestation of sarcoidosis (in older texts it was referred to as lupus pernio, or chilblain lupus).

The course of sarcoid is variable. The lesions may persist for a few months or many years. They may disappear without leaving any residual signs or there may be some scarring.

### Treatment

The only drugs known to have any significant effect on sarcoidosis are corticosteroids. Topically, they have no effect because the lesions are in the dermis and not the epidermis. If the lesions are multiple then systemic corticosteroids have to be given to produce any effect. However, since sarcoid usually runs a fairly protracted course the dangers of long-term systemic corticosteroids must be considered. Generally speaking, if the skin is the only organ involved one could hardly justify the use of these drugs. If the lesions are few, intralesional injection of a corticosteroid may be helpful.

### Purpura and Vasculitis

Purpura is the extravasation of blood from the vessels into the skin or mucous membranes. It presents as a red patch in the skin and has to be distinguished from 'erythema' which is a red patch due to dilatation of the blood vessels in the

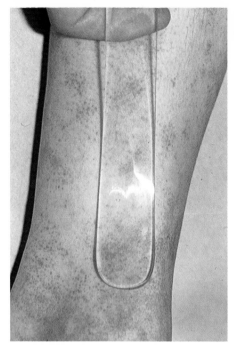

Figure 20.13 *Purpura. The eruption does not blanch on pressure, unlike erythema.*

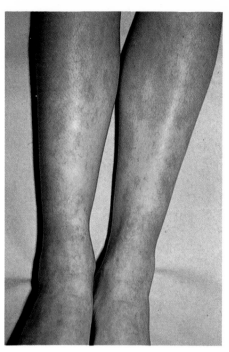

Figure 20.14 *The legs and feet are the commonest sites for purpura.*

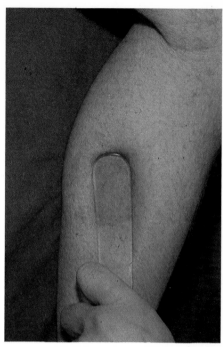

Figure 20.15 *Idiopathic capillaritis. Discoid purpuric eruption which may eventually develop a brown appearance due to haemosiderin.*

skin. If the redness of the skin is due to extravasation of blood (purpura) the colour of the skin will not change on pressure (a glass spatula is best so one can see the result at the same time as applying the pressure) (Figure 20.13). If the redness of the skin is simply due to dilatation of the vessels the skin will blanch.

The purpuric lesion may vary in size from a few mm to a few cm. The commonest site for purpura from whatever cause is the lower limbs (Figure 20.14) because this is the site of maximum venous or back pressure on the capillaries. The causes of purpura are numerous, but it must always be borne in mind that some of the causes are serious disorders and thus all patients must be carefully investigated. Essentially, the aetiology of purpura is due to disorders of the blood or disorders of the vessel wall. The classification of purpura really belongs to the realms of haematology but Table 1 may serve as a useful guide, although it is by no means complete.

Thus, it can be seen that the causes of purpura are numerous and the treatment will depend on the cause. In a book written from the dermatological standpoint it is probably right and justifiable to stress a number of the conditions mentioned above which are most likely to present to the dermatologist.

*Eczema.* It is important to realise that any eczema may be associated with purpuric lesions. This is probably due to a combination of the inflammatory process and trauma (scratching).

*Idiopathic capillaritis.* (Schamberg's disease). The disease is characterised by discoid areas of purpuric lesions on the

Table 1. Classification of purpura.

| Disorders of the blood | Disorders of the blood vessels |
| --- | --- |
| *Deficiencies of Platelets* | Hereditary |
| Idiopathic | Ageing (senile purpura) |
| Leukaemia or carcinomatosis | 'Allergic' (e.g. |
| Vitamin $B_{12}$ deficiency | Henoch-Schönlein) |
| Drugs (e.g. cytotoxics, gold, | Toxic |
| sulphonamides, | Vitamin C deficiency |
| chloramphenicol) | Associated with emboli |
| Systemic lupus erythematosus | (e.g. subacute bacterial |
| | endocarditis) |
| *Disorders of coagulation* | Associated with eczema |
| (other than platelet deficiency) | Idiopathic capillaritis |
| *Diseases producing cryoglobulins and macroglobulins* | |

lower leg (Figure 20.15). Because of the continual leaking of blood into the skin there is frequently residual pigmentation due to haemosiderin. The lesions may spread to involve the thighs and trunk. The lesions are not associated with any internal disorder, the cause is unknown and there is no satisfactory treatment.

*Henoch-Schönlein purpura.* This disease frequently presents to the dermatologist with purpura on the legs and buttocks (Figure 20.16). There may be accompanying nephritis, arthritis and bleeding into the gut. The skin lesions in the

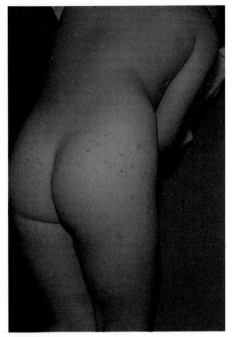

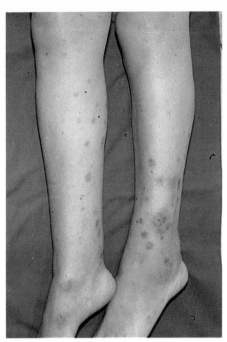

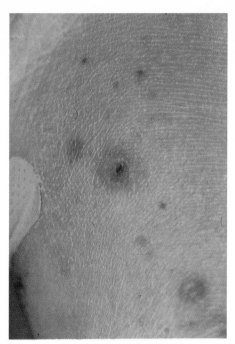

**Figure 20.16** *Henoch-Schönlein purpura. The eruption characteristically appears on the legs and buttocks.*

**Figure 20.17** *Purpuric papules and blisters in cutaneous vasculitis.*

**Figure 20.18** *Haemorrhagic blister in cutaneous vasculitis.*

severe forms may be papules, blisters and necrotic ulcers in addition to the purpura. Henoch-Schönlein purpura is probably what is termed an 'immune-complex' disorder. One of the possible antigens is the streptococcus.

*Vasculitis.* The term is used here to imply damage to arterioles and the small arteries in the skin (cutaneous vasculitis). The disorder usually presents to the dermatologist as multiple purpuric papules and/or blisters if the small superficial vessels are involved (Figure 20.17 and 20.18), or as deeper firm nodules if larger vessels are involved. As with other causes of purpura, the commonest site for cutaneous vasculitis is the lower leg. Occasionally cutaneous vasculitis is associated with a chronic reticular cyanosis on the legs, so-called livedo reticularis (Figure 20.19). The causes of this type of lesion are often similar to those causing purpura. The commonest aetiological factors are 'allergic' (immune-complex, e.g. streptococcal or drugs), toxic (e.g. drugs), and polyarteritis nodosa (cause unknown). The treatment is first to define a cause if possible (e.g. drug or streptococcal infection). If this can be eradicated the disorder is frequently self-limiting. However, if the disorder is continuous, systemic corticosteroids (and possibly immunosuppressive drugs) will be required.

### Lesions in the Skin Due to Internal Malignancy

#### Carcinomata

*Acanthosis nigricans.* In this condition the skin becomes pigmented and thickened (usually due to epidermal hypertrophy) with a rough surface. The commonest sites to be involved are axillae (Figure 20.20), flexures of the limbs, back of the hands and neck. Although acanthosis nigricans is certainly a pointer to internal malignancy, it is not always

so, particularly in obese persons. However, in adults the incidence is so high that one is obliged to screen for carcinomata, especially carcinoma of the stomach.

*Secondary deposits.* Secondary carcinomatous deposits in the skin are relatively rare. When they do occur they present as firm nodules. The diagnosis is established by biopsy.

### Reticuloses

Skin lesions in association with a reticulosis at other sites of

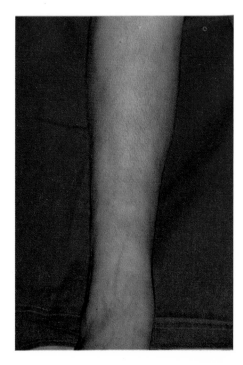

**Figure 20.19**
*Livedo reticularis in polyarteritis nodosa.*

128

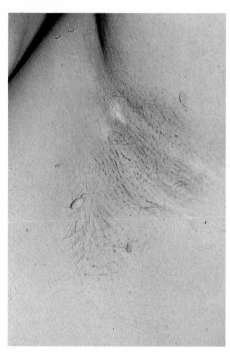

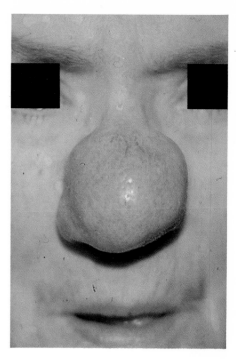

**Figure 20.20** *Thickening and pigmentation of the skin in acanthosis nigricans.*

**Figure 20.22** *Infiltration of the nose with leukaemic cells in chronic lymphatic leukaemia.*

**Figure 20.21** (Below) *Reticulum cell sarcoma. Red, firm, deep nodule in the skin.*

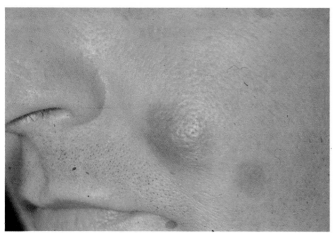

the body is not infrequent. The lesions usually present as firm plaques or nodules. Leukaemia, Hodgkin's disease and sarcomata may all give rise to nodular deposits in the skin (Figure 20.21). Occasionally, the skin lesion is the presenting sign. In chronic lymphatic leukaemia, there is occasionally infiltration of nose (Figure 20.22) and ear lobes with the leukaemic cells, and this presents as a generalised, firm swelling, rather than a solitary nodule.

### Pruritus

Patients who complain of generalised irritation with no obvious skin lesions (other than excoriations) have to be screened for internal disorders. The classical disorder to give rise to this symptom, possibly for years before there are any other signs, is Hodgkin's disease. Pruritus has also been recorded in association with other forms of reticuloses and carcinomata, renal failure and liver disease. In the latter instance, it has been attributed to the high level of bile salts in the skin. This may be lowered by the administration of the resin, cholestyramine. Diabetes mellitus has also been mentioned as a cause of generalised pruritus but this is questionable. The irritation here is usually due to a monilial infection. Pruritus due to psychiatric disorder is well recognised and has to be considered but only after other causes have been excluded.

# 21. Parasitic Infestation and Insect Bites

### Scabies

SCABIES is one of the fairly common disorders seen in a skin clinic. Since it is a disorder with potentially a hundred per cent cure rate with simple treatment this implies that the referring doctor (usually the casualty officer or general practitioner) has missed the diagnosis or has not given the correct medication and instructions to go with it.

### Aetiology

The disorder is caused by an insect (mite—*Sarcoptes scabei var hominis*). The female mite (acarus) which can just be seen by the naked eye, burrows into the keratin layer of the epidermis. In the burrow the mite lays her eggs which hatch after three to four days. Active larvae then emerge from the burrow and invade the adjacent epidermis. After 17 days final male and female adult forms emerge. Copulation then occurs and the gravid female will then wander over the skin surface before burrowing and repeating the cycle. The female may live for six to eight weeks in a burrow and lay up to 50 eggs.

The insect passes from one person to another when there is close bodily contact. The disease is highly contagious and the commonest way to acquire the infection is by sharing a bed with an infected person. Thus invariably there is a positive 'family' history of other members of the family, or a close friend, being similarly affected.

In the early stages of the disorder when the female mite is burrowing in the skin, the patient will probably have no symptoms. However, after the eggs begin to hatch (and usually three to four weeks after the infestation has been acquired) the patient develops a generalised irritating eruption. It is thought that this eruption is due to sensitisation from a substance produced by the mite or possibly by the eggs themselves.

### Clinical Presentation

#### Symptoms

The first symptom of which the patient complains is a generalised irritation when going to bed at night. It appears to be fairly characteristic of scabies that the irritation is worse at night than during the day. Subsequently, the patient will be aware of a rash which may be fairly generalised and the irritation at this stage may also persist during the day.

**Figure 21.1** *The 'burrow' of scabies appears on the palm as a linear, grey, scaly lesion.*

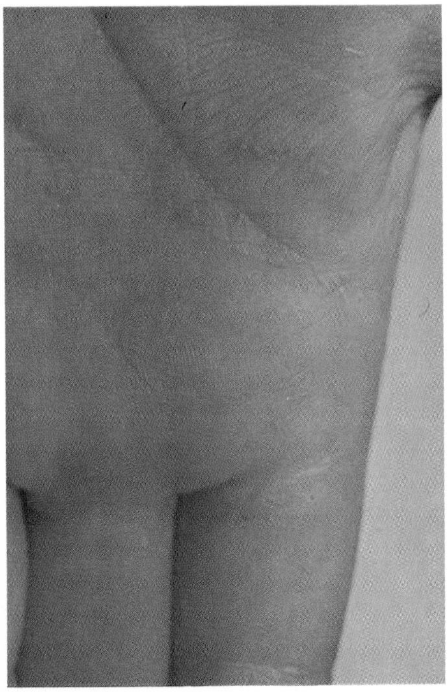

**Figure 21.2** *Two linear, grey, scaly burrows in scabies.*

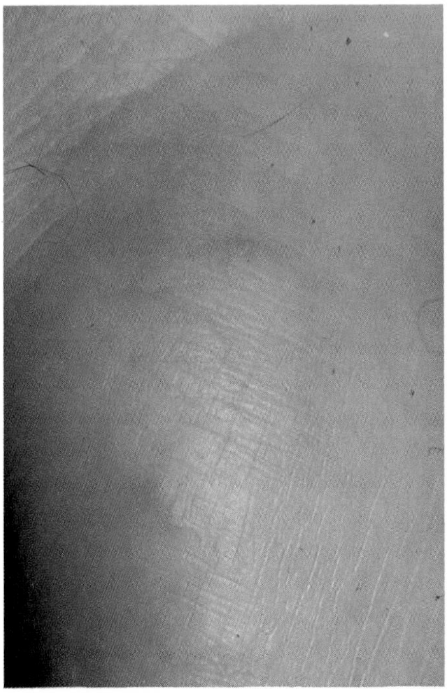

**Figure 21.3** *Small, discrete, scaly areas on the palms suggestive of scabies. Some of the burrows are old and present as red, scaly lesions.*

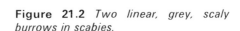

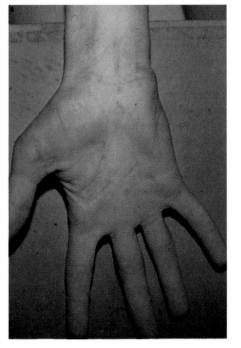

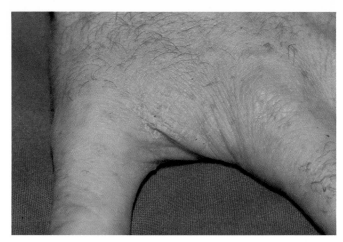

Figure 21.4 *The linear, scaly area, between the thumb and finger is the site of a burrow. This is a common finding in scabies.*

### Signs

The characteristic lesion of scabies infestation is the burrow (Figures 21.1 and 21.2). The classical appearance of a burrow is a greyish linear or slightly curved scaly lesion (Figures 21.1 and 21.2). It is usually 0.5 cm in length and rarely longer than 1.0 cm. Occasionally at one end a small vesicle may be seen. The commonest sites for finding the classical burrow are the palms (Figures 21.1, 21.2 and 21.3), between the fingers (Figures 21.4 and 21.5) and wrists. Not infrequently the classical burrow is not found, but superficial, scaly lesions (the same size as burrows) are found between the fingers (Figure 21.4) or on the palms (Figure 21.3). The lesions sometimes become secondarily infected and present as crusted lesions (Figure 21.5) or pustules.

Although the acarus may 'burrow' at other sites, notably the breasts (in females), the external genitalia (in males) (Figures 21.6, 21.7 and 21.8), on the buttocks (Figure 21.9) and the umbilicus, the classical burrow may not be seen at these sites. The lesions may present as firm, deep, red papules (Figures 21.6, 21.7 and 21.8). There may be some superficial scaling or excoriation. This type of lesion on the male genitalia and buttocks is often as diagnostic as the typical burrow on the hands. In infants under the age of a year a common site for the mite's burrow is the soles of the feet. The lesions may present here as small blisters.

By the time the patient seeks medical advice there is usually a generalised eruption on the trunk and limbs but the head is never involved except in children under two years of age. The generalised eruption takes the form of excoriated papular urticarial lesions (Figure 21.10). In children the eruption on the trunk (Figure 21.11), and particularly around and in the axillae (Figure 21.12), presents as firm red papules. These lesions are fairly characteristic of scabies. The generalised eruption in scabies is thought to be an allergic reaction to the contents of the burrow whether they be from the mite, eggs or excreta of the mite.

It should be remembered that because of the intense irritation and subsequent scratching there is frequently secondary bacterial infection which presents as impetigo and boils and destroys the typical structure, and therefore appearances, of the burrows.

The most satisfactory way to confirm the diagnosis is to demonstrate the presence of the acarus (Figure 21.13) in a burrow on the hands or a papule on the male genitalia or buttocks. This is best done by gently scraping the burrow with a blunt scalpel blade and examining the contents under a low power microscope field. Even if the acarus itself is not

**Figure 21.5** Crusted and scabbed lesions between the fingers in scabies. These are excoriated and infected burrows.

**Figure 21.6** Papules on the penis in scabies. Some linear scaling is present.

**Figures 21.7** Numerous, firm, deep papules on the penis and scrotum. These lesions are fairly characteristic of scabies.

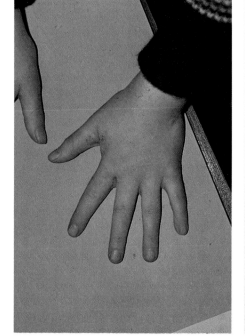

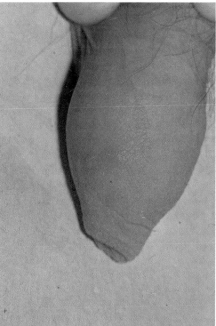

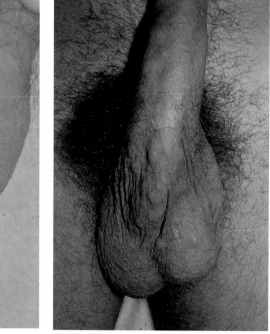

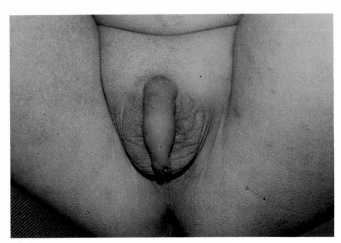

**Figure 21.8** *Papules on the genitalia. In a child the lesions may persist for months after treatment.*

seen, eggs may be found. From the practical point of view, however, in general practice when a microscope is not available, the typical clinical appearances and a positive family history are usually all that is required to make the diagnosis.

### Norwegian Scabies

This form of scabies is rare and has a completely different clinical picture from the disorder described above. It usually occurs in the elderly or in patients with mental deficiency living in institutions. The typical clinical appearance is a generalised scaly redness of the skin with thick, hyperkeratotic crusting on the hands, feet and elbows. It is important to be aware of this condition as it is frequently misdiagnosed as a generalised eczema and thus mistreated. Norwegian scabies is contagious and is often only diagnosed

when a nurse or some other person looking after the patient develops scabies. The reason for the difference of the clinical appearance in Norwegian scabies from that in 'ordinary' scabies is unknown but must be due to host factors as the parasite is the same.

### Treatment and Management

Patients often arrive in a skin clinic from a general practitioner with the correct diagnosis of scabies having been made, but treatment having failed. There are two very important points in the treatment of scabies. First, the lotion must be applied to *all* the skin surface from the neck to the soles of the feet and, second, the whole household (and boyfriends and girlfriends) must all be treated simultaneously. If these two simple rules are observed it is usually immaterial which 'anti-scabies' preparation is used. Benzyl benzoate application B.P., gamma benzene hexachloride lotion 1 per cent and crotamiton lotion 10 per cent are all effective.

The treatment is carried out as follows:—a) The patient has a bath and then dries himself. b) The lotion is then applied to the whole body (with cotton wool), apart from the head. c) The lotion should be applied again 24 hours later. d) Twenty-four hours after the second application the patient has another bath. e) The bed sheets and underwear should be changed, but it is not necessary to send outer clothing or blankets to the laundry or dry cleaning firms.

It is important to tell the patient that the irritation may persist for a week or two after treatment (this is due to an allergic reaction, although the mite has been killed). If patients are not told that the irritation may persist they usually continue to anoint themselves and produce an

**Figure 21.9** *Firm, red, discrete papules on the buttocks; a common and typical finding in scabies.*

**Figure 21.10** *The generalised eruption of scabies is papular and urticarial and excoriations are frequently present.*

**Figure 21.11** *Large, deep papules and nodules on the trunk in scabies in an infant. This type of eruption is usually only seen in infants.*

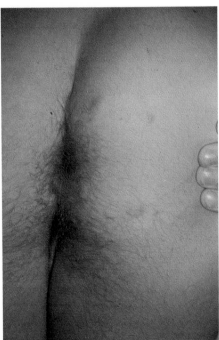

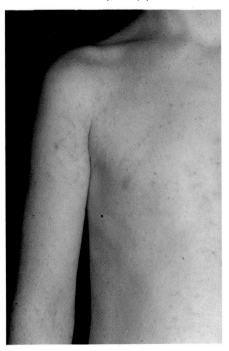

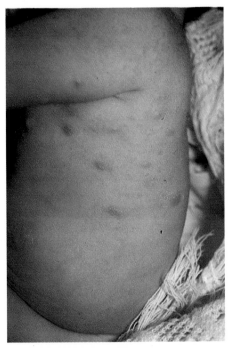

132

irritant eczema (particularly if they are using benzyl benzoate). Thus, although cured of their scabies, they will continue to itch because of an iatrogenic eczema.

It is also important to realise that the papular lesions on the genitalia and around the axillae, particularly in children, may persist for many months after successful treatment. The papules represent an 'immunological' reaction in the skin with chronic inflammatory cells and they do not disperse for a considerable length of time.

### Pediculosis (Lice)

Clinically, pediculosis may present as three distinct entities depending on the species and varieties of the louse.

#### Pediculosis Capitis (Head Lice)

This is a contagious disorder seen predominantly in children. The main symptom is pruritus of the scalp due to bites from the insect. Because of the irritation there is continual scratching and this not infrequently becomes secondarily infected by bacteria. Thus, if a child is brought to the clinic complaining of scalp irritation or with impetigo of the scalp and excoriations are present, it is most important to think of head lice as a cause of the symptoms and signs.

The characteristic feature of head lice is nits on the hair shaft. The mature form of insect has a relatively short life but the female lays numerous eggs close to the scalp surface which develop into nits. Clinically, they are small white specks (Figure 21.14) firmly attached to the hair shaft. The commonest site is the hair behind the ears but any part of the scalp hair may be involved. The nits are approximately 0.5 mm in length and have to be distinguished from scales in the hair from seborrhoeic eczema (dandruff). Nits are firmly attached to the hair and cannot be brushed off, whereas scales from dandruff can easily be removed. The nits can sometimes be slid along the hair shaft. If a microscope is available the diagnosis can be easily established by cutting off a hair with a nit attached and examining it under a low power field (Figure 21.15). The nit will be seen as an oval structure firmly attached to the hair by a sheath which completely encases the shaft. Very occasionally the actual insect may be found in the scalp and is visible with the naked eye.

#### Treatment

The present treatment for head lice is either gamma benzene hexachloride solution 1 per cent or malathion solution 0.5 per cent. The former is used as a lotion after the hair has been washed and should be left on the scalp for 24 hours. The malathion is applied directly to the scalp and hair and is left for 12 hours. After the use of either preparation the scalp is shampooed and the hair is combed with a fine comb whilst wet. The treatment is repeated after a week. It is probably advisable to treat all members of the household, particularly children, at the same time, even if they have no symptoms. Nits can be removed even though they are not visible by means of a 'nit comb'— a very fine metal comb. If this cannot be obtained from a chemist, some public health departments have a supply.

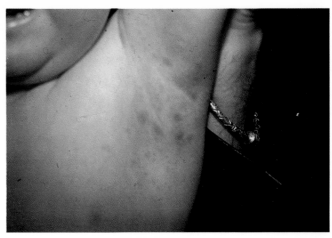

**Figure 21.12** *A common site for the large papular type of eruption in scabies is in and around the axilla.*

**Figure 21.13** *The acarus isolated from a burrow, viewed in the low power field of a microscope.*

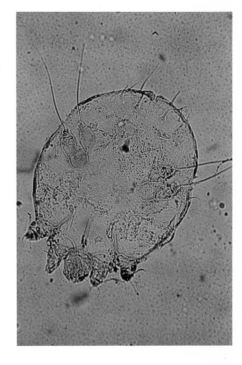

**Figure 21.14** *Nits presenting as small white 'dots' on the hairs of the scalp. They have to be distinguished from the scales of dandruff (seborrhoeic eczema).*

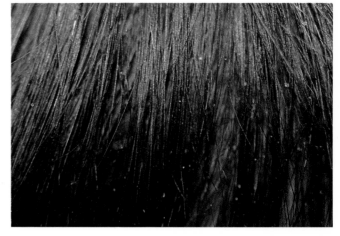

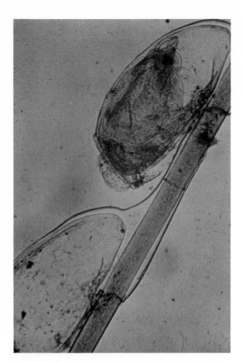

Figure 21.15
*Nit of louse attached to a hair, as seen in low power field of microscope.*

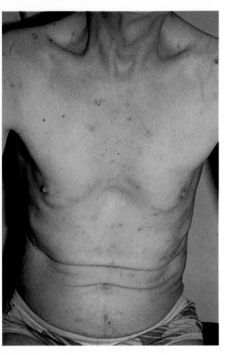

Figure 21.16
*Excoriations and excoriated papules due to pediculosis corporis. The commonest site affected is the trunk.*

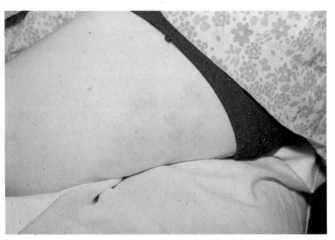

## Pediculosis Corporis (Body Lice)

This has become a very rare affliction and is usually only seen in persons whose personal hygiene is very poor. It is now usually encountered in the 'tramp' who arrives at a casualty department for one reason or another. The body louse is rarely found on the skin as it lives in seams of clothing and leaves only for 'meals'. The nits are firmly attached to the fibres of clothing. Thus, if pediculosis corporis is suspected it is important to examine the clothes, particularly the underclothes, for the parasite which is visible to the naked eye.

The characteristic skin lesion resulting from a bite is a small red macule. Occasionally there is a papule with a central haemorrhagic punctum. The most frequent sites for the bites are on the trunk. There is intense irritation and thus on examination the most obvious features are extensive and severe excoriations (Figure 21.16) and not the individual bites. There is frequently secondary bacterial infection. In severe and longstanding infestation the skin becomes pigmented, dry, scaly and eczematised and there are scars from previous excoriations. These features are sometimes referred to as 'vagabond's disease'.

### Treatment

The skin should be treated with 1 per cent gamma benzene hexachloride cream. The clothes must also be treated with gamma benzene hexachloride lotion or powder and sent for laundering.

## Pediculosis Pubis (Pubic Lice)

The principal site of involvement is the pubic hair but the lice may involve other areas and the nits have been known to become attached to axillary and body hair (other than pubic), eyelashes and eyebrows. The main symptom is pruritus produced by bites from the insect. Thus, on examination, there are excoriations and possibly secondary bacterial infection. The mature parasite is often visible and nits are attached to the hair shafts.

### Treatment

This is either 1 per cent benzene hexachloride lotion, which should be left on the affected areas for 24 hours, or 0.5 per cent malathion solution which should be left on the affected hairs for 12 hours.

## Insect Bites (Papular Urticaria)

The typical skin lesion produced by an insect bite, i.e. an urticarial lesion with a central punctum and surrounding flare (Figure 21.17), is easily recognised as such by lay persons. However, occasionally there is a different type of clinical response and this results in the person seeking medical advice. It is not possible to say which particular insect produces the lesions seen most frequently in a skin clinic but undoubtedly there are many different species, e.g.

**Figure 21.17** (Left) *An urticarial lesion with a central (haemorrhagic) punctum. The typical lesion produced by insect bites.*

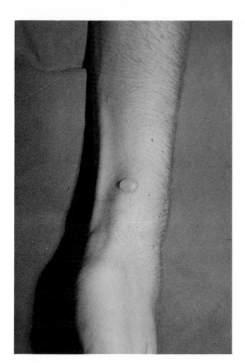

**Figure 21.18**
*Large tense blister caused by an insect bite.*

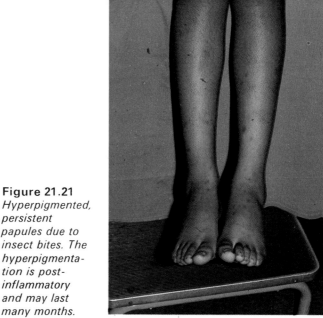

**Figure 21.21**
*Hyperpigmented, persistent papules due to insect bites. The hyperpigmentation is post-inflammatory and may last many months.*

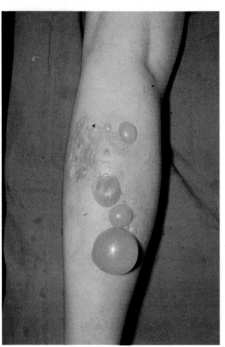

**Figure 21.19**
*Acute inflammatory response with large blisters due to insect bites.*

fleas, flies, mosquitoes, bedbugs, etc. There are two main clinical patterns most commonly seen in a skin clinic.

First, there may be an acute urticarial eruption with subsequent blister formation (Figures 21.18 and 21.19), the blisters being a few cm in diameter on occasions. On account of the size of the blisters the patient seeks medical advice. The lesions are usually present on the exposed areas, e.g. below the knees (Figure 21.19), forearms (Figure 21.20) and hands and, occasionally, the face.

The second type of clinical presentation is persistent papules, most commonly seen in children, on the arms and legs (Figures 21.20 and 21.21), but occasionally on the trunk. The papules are usually 2–3 mm in diameter and a clue to the diagnosis is often present in the form of a central punctum. In the early stages there is a central weal, flare and central punctum which is characteristic of insect bites. It is the persistence of the lesions beyond a few days which confuses doctor and patient and results in referral to a dermatologist. The cause for the persistence of the lesion is not certain but is probably due to an altered immuno-logical response on the part of the patient. The papules are due to a persistent cellular infiltrate and may take months to disappear. The lesions are always discrete with normal skin in between and there is sometimes residual scarring. In negroes this type of lesion invariably leads to post-inflam-matory hyperpigmentation (Figure 21.21), which may persist for a few months, and this is another cause for referral to a skin clinic. The hyperpigmentation eventually fades.

### Treatment and Management

The treatment of the acute blistering eruption is sympto-matic with systemic antihistamines. The lesions usually

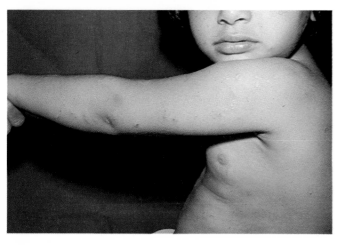

**Figure 21.20** (Left) *Small, persistent papules due to insect bites.*

settle within a few days. Dry non-adhesive dressings may be required when the blisters burst. If the eruption is very acute and widespread a short course of systemic steroids should be given.

In the second type of eruption, with persistent, small papules it is often very difficult to convince parents that the lesions on the child are due to insect bites. There are probably two reasons for this. First, this type of lesion with its persistence is not what the parent associates with insect bites and, secondly, they cannot think of the source of the insects. If there is an animal pet at home then this is frequently the source but various types of insect may live in the furniture or in the gardens of those patients who are affected. The main problem is often not so much the source of the insects as the altered immunological response of the patient. Treatment is often unsatisfactory. If the source can be identified, i.e., a domestic animal, this should be treated if necessary with the help of a vet. Animals are often re-infested from other animals. Insecticide powders containing DDT have now been taken off the market, but powders containing pyrethrum are effective in treating furniture etc. Insect repellents (in the form of dimethylphthalate) are of limited help. Systemic antihistamines may relieve irritation but do not appear to induce the lesions to resolve more quickly. Fortunately, the majority of children appear to lose this hypersensitive response to insect bites in due course.

# 22. Photosensitivity and Tropical Infections

W ITH the advent of air travel and affluence many more people are travelling abroad and patients are now presenting with disorders attributable to different climates, and doctors must be aware of these problems.

The term 'photosensitivity' is used to imply an abnormal response to ultraviolet irradiation. It has to be distinguished from ordinary 'sunburn' which occurs in caucasians after prolonged exposure to sunlight (particularly strong sunlight) in those whose skin has not adapted to the sun by pigmentation, i.e. usually the first day of a holiday. As such, 'sunburn' and the long term effects of ultraviolet light on the skin are 'normal' responses in the caucasian but will be discussed in some detail as they may present as a medical problem.

## Normal Reactions to Sunlight
### Sunburn

This is by far the commonest adverse reaction produced by sunlight. The three important factors which determine sunburn are the degree of pigmentation prior to going into the sunlight (fair skin persons are more at risk), the length of time exposed, and the strength of the sun (the more vertical the rays the more damaging they are to the skin). Sunburn is characterised by a biphasic erythema response. The initial erythema occurs during exposure and disappears shortly thereafter. The delayed erythema usually begins 2–4 hours after exposure and reaches a peak in approximately 15 hours and persists for up to 48 hours. This stage is accompanied by pain and discomfort if the erythema has been severe.

**Figure 22.1** *Actinic lentigos. Hyperpigmented macules caused by many years exposure to sunlight.*

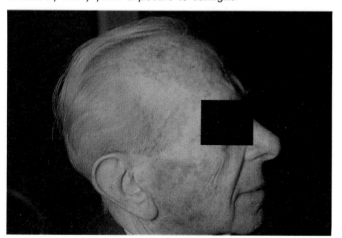

Very occasionally there may be oedema of the skin and blister formation. The erythema stage is followed by peeling of the skin.

The cause of sunburn is that of a 'phototoxic' reaction in the skin. The energy in the sun's rays causes the release of certain chemicals in the skin which accounts for the inflammatory response. The sunburn reaction in normal subjects is caused by rays of a certain wavelength (290–320 nm which constitute short wave ultra-violet light, UVB).

### Treatment and Management

Once the patient has developed 'sunburn', treatment is symptomatic. Further exposure to sunlight must be avoided until the erythema subsides. Topical steroid creams may diminish the inflammatory response. For a short duration (2 to 3 days) one of the strong steroid preparations should be used. A cream-based preparation should be prescribed as the cream itself may have a soothing effect and should be applied 3 to 4 times a day. Mild analgesics and sedatives can be given if the patient is in severe discomfort.

Patients with fair skin should be warned not to stay ex-

**Figure 22.2** *Actinic lentigos. Hyperpigmented macules in a young woman who lived in Northern Australia.*

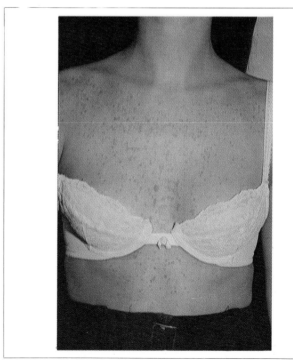

posed in the sunlight for long periods and given sunscreen preparations to use. At the present time the most effective preparations are para-amino benzoic acid and the ester amyl dimethyl aminobenzoate in alcoholic solutions. These preparations should be applied each morning before the patient goes in to the sunlight. The protection lasts for approximately eight hours.

### Chronic Effects of Sunlight

These are also within normal limits for caucasians who live in 'sunny' climates. The changes vary with the degree of pigmentation (and thus protection) and the duration of exposure. The changes include wrinkling due to damage to the elastic tissue, atrophy, hyperpigmented macules (lentigos) (Figures 22.1 and 22.2), telangiectasia and actinic keratoses. In addition, ultra-violet irradiation is carcinogenic. Basal cell and squamous cell carcinomata are most commonly found on exposed areas and are more common in white persons living in South Africa and Australia than those living in England.

### Abnormal Reactions to Sunlight —Photosensitivity

These may occur in the following three situations:

(1) When a known substance in the skin, either from internal causes or applied externally, 'sensitises' the skin.

(2) In disorders resulting in deficient protection.

(3) With no known cause (at present) for the reaction.

### Known Photosensitisers

*Porphyria.* This is a disease in which there is abnormal porphyrin metabolism with resulting increase of circulating porphyrins which become deposited in the skin. Some of the porphyrins cause photosensitivity. The classification of porphyria is unsatisfactory. From a simple clinical point of view, porphyria could be classified as those cases in which the abnormal porphyrin metabolism is in a) the bone marrow, b) the liver or c) at both sites. Alternatively, porphyria can be classified as that involving photosensitivity and that not. The photosensitivity depends on which particular porphyrins are produced and this depends on the basic biochemical abnormality present. One type of porphyria associated with light sensitivity has recently been shown to involve abnormal iron metabolism. It is thought possible that an increase in the absorption of iron occurs and a raised serum iron is frequently found. The cause for this abnormal iron metabolism is unknown. The skin lesions may present as an acute erythema or blisters in the light-exposed areas. The former is usually present in young children and the latter in adults. There is increased skin fragility and minor trauma produces blisters which break and form scabs (Figures 22.3 and 22.4). Scarring in the light-exposed areas is a common finding. In adults there is occasionally increased pigmentation (Figure 22.5) and excess hair growth.

**Figure 22.5** (Right) *Increased pigmentation of the skin which may occur in porphyria.*

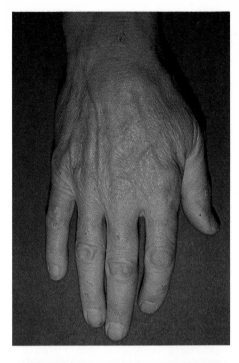

**Figure 22.3**
*Scabbed lesions on the backs of the hands following minor trauma in porphyria.*

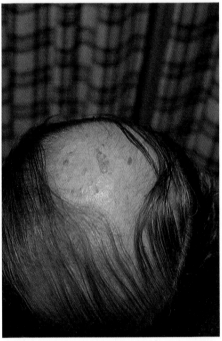

**Figure 22.4**
*Ruptured blisters and scarring in the bald area of the scalp due to exposure to sunlight in porphyria.*

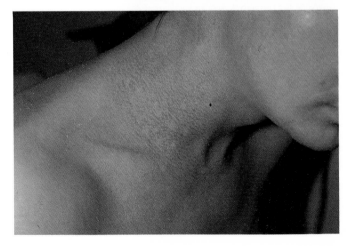

*Systemic drugs.* A number of drugs taken orally cause photosensitivity. The commonest drugs to elicit this response are the sulphonamides (Figure 22.6), sulphonyl-ureas, tetracyclines (Figure 22.7), phenothiazines (particularly chlorpromazine), thiazide diuretics and nalidixic acid. The type of rash produced is usually an acute erythema (Figure 22.7) sometimes with accompanying blisters and subsequent peeling of the skin. It should be remembered that any drug can cause any rash and photosensitisation may be the end result.

*Topical photosensitisers.* Probably the most common topical photosensitisers are the essential oils in cosmetics. The one most frequently incriminated is oil of bergamot. This may cause acute erythema (Figure 22.8), blisters and subsequent pigmentation (Figure 22.9). Occasionally, only the excess pigmentation results. The commonest site for this pattern of reaction is the sides of the neck resulting from perfumes applied behind the ears and sides of the neck. Other topical photosensitisers are chemicals from plants, tar preparations (Figure 22.10), halogenated salicylanides (which have been used in soaps and deodorants) and a substance called bithionol which has been used in shampoos.

## Adverse Reactions from Deficient Protection

As has already been stated, melanin pigmentation offers protection from the damaging effects of the sun's rays. Thus, in disorders in which melanin formation is deficient or impaired there will be abnormal reactions to sunlight. These conditions include albinism, oculo-cutaneous albinism, vitiligo, phenylketonuria and affect persons with fair hair and light complexions. There is a rare condition called xeroderma pigmentosa in which there is an abnormality in the repair of the skin cells' DNA following damage after exposure to sunlight. This failure to repair DNA results in malignant skin conditions at a very early age, usually in childhood.

## Photosensitivity Reactions with Unknown Causes

*Systemic lupus erythematosus.* Patients with this condition frequently develop an erythematous eruption in the exposed areas, particularly the face. The classical distribution is the nose and cheeks—so called butterfly rash. The eruption is usually an intense erythema (Figure 22.11) but urticarial and vesicular eruptions have also been reported.

*Solar urticaria and polymorphic light eruption.* As the name implies the predominant skin lesion in some patients on exposure to sunlight is urticarial. This type of lesion usually develops on the exposed areas after a few minutes of exposure to sunlight. The urticarial lesions usually subside within an hour after exposure. In the 'delayed type' of reaction there may be erythematous, blistering or urticarial lesions developing from a few hours to a few days after

**Figure 22.8** (Right) *Photosensitivity due to essential oils in perfume.*

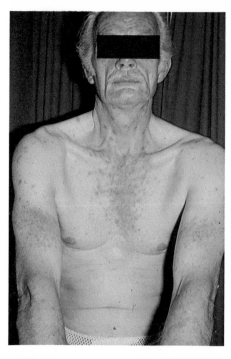

**Figure 22.6**
*Erythema multiforme produced in light-exposed areas by sulphonamides. A few lesions are present in the unexposed areas.*

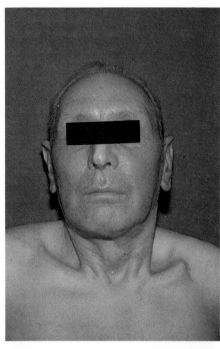

**Figure 22.7**
*Confluent erythema and scaling due to photosensitivity from tetra-cyclines.*

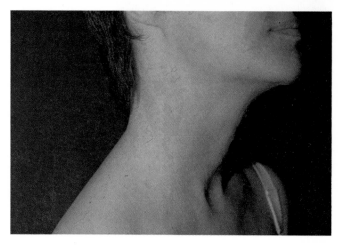

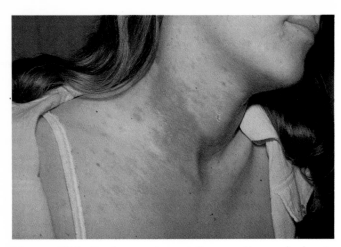

**Figure 22.9** *Persistent pigmentation on the neck due to photosensitivity from perfume.*

exposure to sunlight. This type of response has been termed the polymorphic light eruption (Figures 22.12 and 22.13).

### Treatment and Management of Photosensitivity

In the first instance it is most important to enquire if the patient has taken or is taking any drugs which are possible photosensitisers. Secondly, enquiry should be made as to whether cosmetics or any creams or lotions containing possible photosensitisers have been used. Enquiry should also be made about possible contact with plants. Unless an obvious cause for the photosensitivity is found, all patients should be screened for porphyria and systemic lupus erythematosus, the former by examination of blood, faeces and urine for excess porphyrins; the latter by examination of the blood for 'LE cells' and anti-nuclear antibodies. If exogenous photosensitisers are considered likely it is possible to carry out photo-patch tests with the suspected substances. The chemicals are applied to the back and then irradiated by ultraviolet light.

Treatment of photosensitivity will, to a certain extent, depend on the underlying cause. If it is due to systemic drugs or applied substances these should obviously be avoided if possible. If the patient has porphyria, then further investigations will be required to determine if they have the type associated with abnormal iron metabolism. In light sensitive porphyria associated with raised serum iron, the severity of the light eruption can be decreased and even the lesions prevented by lowering the serum iron by venepuncture. If lupus erythematosus is found then further investigations will be required before deciding on the appropriate treatment.

Sunscreen preparations are of some help in preventing or alleviating the eruptions caused by light. The chemical light screening agents para-aminobenzoic acid and amyl dimethylbenzoate in alcoholic solution are cosmetically acceptable and easy to use, but they are only effective in screening out short wave ultra-violet light (290–320 nm). The only effective agents for screening out long wave ultra-violet light (320–400 nm) and visible light (740 nm) are physical agents. That used most often is titanium dioxide. Colouring agents are added to it to make it cosmetically acceptable for patient use. Thus in order to advise patients about which preparation to use it is necessary to know which part of the spectrum is responsible for the rash. It is possible to test patients with the appropriate apparatus, but there are not many centres with the necessary equipment, and in practice it is often a matter of trial and error to determine which sunscreen will be effective. The eruption in porphyria,

**Figure 22.10** *An acute eczematous reaction due to photosensitivity following use of a tar preparation.*

**Figure 22.11** *Erythema and scaling in the exposed areas in systemic lupus erythematosus.*

**Figure 22.12** *Erythematous papules and vesicles in polymorphic light eruption.*

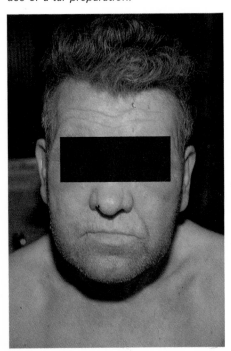
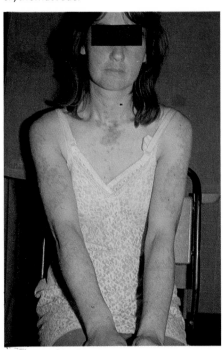
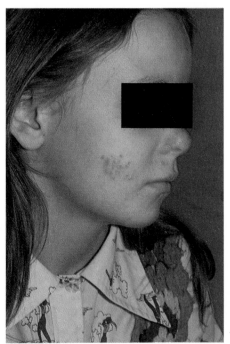

photosensitive eczema, drug eruptions and polymorphic light eruption is usually caused by long wave ultra-violet light or visible light, so chemical sunscreens will be of little or no use.

The antimalarial drug chloroquin has been used for many years in the treatment of solar urticaria and polymorphic light eruption, but its use cannot be recommended because of possible damage to the retina even if it is given for only a short period. Systemic steroids in moderate doses e.g. 20 mg prednisone daily can sometimes completely suppress the eruption of solar urticaria and polymorphic light eruption. Obviously systemic steroids should be used with caution and only for short periods. Potent topical corticosteroid preparations are helpful in controlling the eczematous reactions of polymorphic light eruption and systemic antihistamines in treating the urticarial reactions.

## Tropical Infections

### Leprosy

This is still an extremely rare condition to be seen in a skin clinic in Britain. However, because of the immigration into this country of persons from places where leprosy is endemic, a few patients with the disorder are encountered and thus the physician must be aware of the disease and its presenting symptoms and signs.

Leprosy occurs in tropical climates but is most common in the sub-continent of India, West Africa, South China and Burma. The disease is caused by an organism *Mycobacterium leprae* but evidence is now accumulating that the disease process is influenced by immunological responses of the host. The skin, nerves, reticulo-endothelial system, mucous membranes, eyes and testes may be affected by the disease process. The classification of leprosy is unsatisfactory at the present time but for clinical purposes it is usually divided into:

a) *Lepromatous leprosy.* In this type there is little immunity to the organism and thus the lesions contain many organisms. The course of the disease is often progressive.

b) *Tuberculoid leprosy.* Organisms are rare. Resistance to the organisms is high and the course is benign with a tendency to spontaneous cure.

c) *Intermediate or dimorphous leprosy.* This is applied to a group of patients who do not have the classical features of either lepromatous or tuberculoid leprosy. It appears that in this group resistance is uncertain at first and the clinical course may follow either that of lepromatous or tuberculoid leprosy.

*Lepromatous leprosy.* The skin lesions have indistinct borders and there is a diffuse infiltration of the skin (Figures 22.14 and 22.15) and mucous membranes. Frequently, nodules develop in the skin particularly on the face and ears (Figure 22.14). The nasal mucosa is invariably affected and there is eventually destruction of the nasal septum and subsequent facial deformity. The skin may eventually ulcerate. The eye is also frequently affected. Erythema

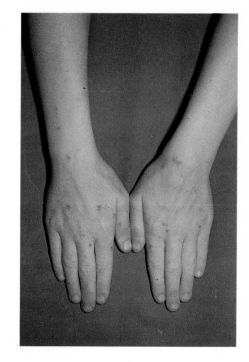

**Figure 22.13**
*Scabbed lesions on the backs of the hands in polymorphic light eruption.*

**Figure 22.14**
(Below)
*Lepromatous leprosy. Infiltrated nodules on the face and ears.*

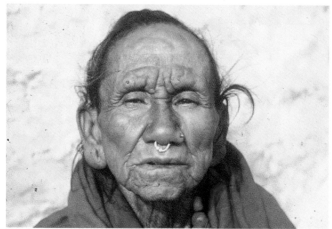

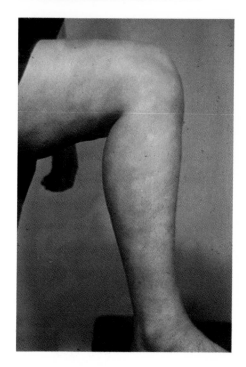

**Figure 22.15**
*Numerous infiltrated plaques on the leg in dimorphous leprosy.*

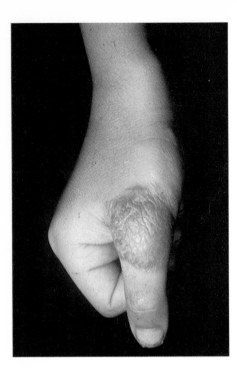

**Figure 22.16**
*Infiltrated plaque on the hand in tuberculoid leprosy.*

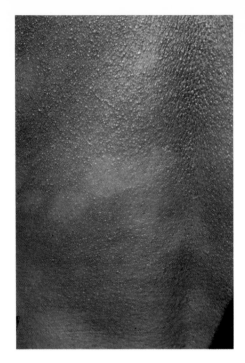

**Figure 22.18**
*Hypopigmented areas on the back in dimorphous leprosy.*

**Figure 22.17** *Large infiltrated plaque and small nodule on the face in dimorphous leprosy. The posterior auricular nerve is thickened and visible on the side of the neck.*

**Figure 22.19** *Hypopigmented areas on the back in tuberculoid leprosy.*

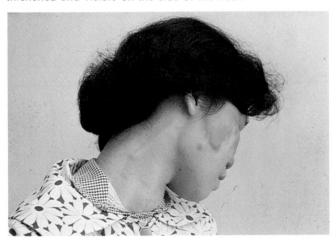

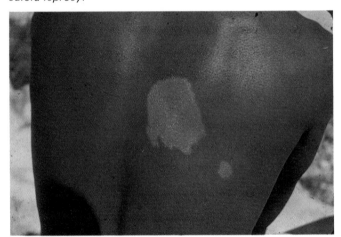

nodosum lesions frequently occur in lepromatous leprosy at the start of treatment with sulphones.

*Tuberculoid leprosy.* The lesions often present as infiltrated plaques, frequently on the face (Figures 22.16 and 22.17). The lesions are often hypopigmented and this may be the first sign which causes the patient to consult a doctor (Figures 22.18 and 22.19). The lesions are often anaesthetic and are hypohydrotic due to nerve involvement. Polyneuropathy is common in all types of leprosy and palpating the ulnar, lateral popliteal and posterior auricular nerves (Figure 22.17) to feel if they are thickened is often used as a clinical diagnostic aid. Because of the neuropathy there may be atrophy of the muscles and weakness. In addition, because of sensory loss, ulceration of the skin from trauma is common. Gross destruction of the tissue also occurs due to trophic changes which accompany severe neuropathies.

The diagnosis of leprosy is made on the histological features of a biopsy of a skin lesion and possibly finding the organism on nasal smears.

### Treatment

The commonest drug used in the treatment of leprosy in the past has been dapsone but many other drugs, including thiabutazine, clofazimine, and rifampicin, are now employed and the choice is usually left to the leprologists.

### Yaws

Although this is a disorder of tropical countries, because of immigration from the West Indies to Britain, and air travel generally, some knowledge and awareness of the disorder is important.

The disease is caused by a spirochaete, *Treponema per-*

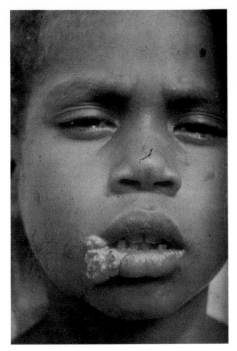

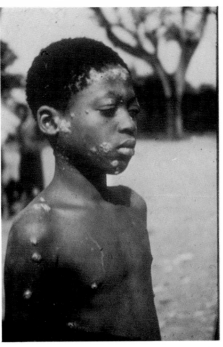

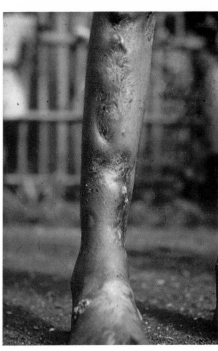

**Figure 22.20** *Primary yaws. Large papillomatous lesion.*

**Figure 22.21** *Widespread eruption in secondary yaws. The lesions may be papular or granulomatous with ulceration.*

**Figure 22.22** *Tertiary yaws. Severe scarring following ulceration of the legs.*

*tenue* and is indistinguishable on serological tests from *Treponema pallidum* which causes syphilis. Like syphilis, yaws has three stages. The primary lesion develops 3 to 4 weeks after the organism has entered the skin. The lesion begins as a small papule which then enlarges (Figure 22.20) or other papules develop around the original lesion and the whole area becomes a confluent crusted lesion. Approximately 2–3 months later (in some cases longer) the secondary stage commences. This is usually a widespread papular eruption, but granulomatous lesions which ulcerate may also occur (Figure 22.21). The lesions fade and do not leave scars. The lesions in the secondary stage may persist for many weeks or months. The tertiary stage of yaws begins after a few years. The skin and bones are the organs most commonly affected. The lesions include gummatous nodules, spreading ulcers (Figure 22.22), periostitis, tenosynovitis and hyperkeratosis of the palms and soles. Unlike syphilis, the heart and nervous system are not involved.

Treatment with penicillin is simple.

### Cutaneous Leishmaniasis

Again, because holidays in the southern Mediterranean countries and the Middle East are now far more common, it is important to be aware of this condition. The disease is also endemic in Africa, Asia, Central and South America.

Cutaneous leishmaniasis is caused by a protozoon. The organism affects animals and is carried by the sandfly.

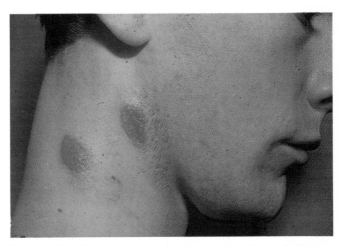

**Figure 22.23** *Cutaneous leishmaniasis. Red, infiltrated plaques on the neck.*

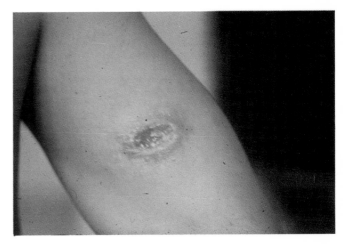

**Figure 22.24** (Right) *Cutaneous leishmaniasis. Ulcerated lesion on the elbow.*

143

## Clinical Features

The incubation period varies from weeks to months, thus, although the patient may not have been abroad for the last few months, the disease should still be considered if the lesion is suggestive. The lesion most commonly occurs on the exposed areas, e.g. face, neck or arms. It begins as a small papule which enlarges to form a nodule or plaque (Figure 22.23). It may become scaly and ulcerate ('Oriental Sore') (Figure 22.24).

After a few months the lesion frequently heals spontaneously leaving a depressed scar. As in the case of patients with leprosy, it is thought that the course of the disease may well depend on the host's immune responses at the time of the infection.

The diagnosis is made by biopsy and by finding the parasite on smears from the ulcer.

## Treatment

Often none is required as the lesion is self-healing. In resistant or recurrent cases some success has been reported using intralesional and systemic steroids combined with injections of organic antimony.

# 23. Hereditary Disorders and Dermatitis Artefacta

## Hereditary Disorders

THE diseases to be discussed in this chapter are relatively rare, but specific, disease entities in which there are known genetic factors involved in their causation, whether the mode of inheritance be dominant or recessive. When discussing hereditary disorders it must be kept in mind that many of the commoner skin diseases such as atopic eczema and psoriasis also have strong genetic backgrounds, and a number of the rarer disorders such as familial hyperlipoproteinaemia, epidermolysis bullosa and xerodermia pigmentosa have already been described in other chapters. It is probable that many skin diseases are partly genetically determined and, thus, to use the title 'hereditary disorders' for a few specific diseases is somewhat misleading. It should also be stressed that the term 'genetic disease' should not be used synonymously with 'congenital disease' as many genetic diseases are not present at birth but appear in childhood or even adult life.

## Ichthyosis

This is a disorder of keratinisation. There are a number of clinical varieties of ichthyosis. In the commonest form the skin is dry, scaly and slightly thickened and often gives the appearance of having cracked (Figures 23.1 and 23.2). Frequently the skin is darker than normal (Figures 23.1 and 23.2) and the patients are often accused of not washing. Ichthyosis does not always involve all the skin. It is commoner on the extensor surfaces and the flexures of the limbs are frequently spared (Figure 23.3), which is the opposite distribution to that of atopic eczema. There are many other clinical varieties of inherited abnormalities of keratinisation. The commonest is hyperkeratinisation around the hair follicles on the outer aspect of the upper arms, buttocks, and front of the thighs. The lesions present as small, rough papules. Ichthyosis may or may not be present at birth. When present at birth it is usual for all the skin to be involved, and the skin dries soon after birth and presents with large 'cracks', the so-called 'collodion' baby. Another, very rare form of ichthyosis is greatly thickened and ridged keratin associated with blisters and erythema of the skin. In this form, the disorder is most marked in the flexures of the limbs.

Ichthyosis is usually more pronounced in childhood and

**Figure 23.1** *Dry, scaly hyperpigmented skin in ichthyosis.*

**Figure 23.2** *Hyperpigmented, scaly skin in ichthyosis. The skin has the appearance of having 'cracked'.*

**Figure 23.3** *Sparing of the flexures in the common form of ichthyosis.*

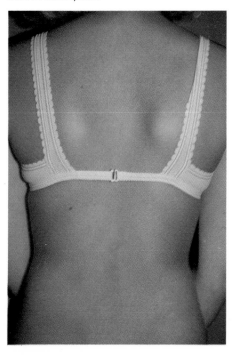

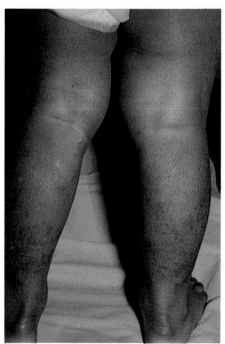

tends to improve spontaneously in early adult life. Keratin bonding and thus skin cracking is directly related to the air temperature. When the temperature is reduced, skin tends to crack and thus ichthyosis is worse in winter and cold climates and improves when the air temperature rises. Thus, patients who go on holiday to a country with a hot climate often have a dramatic improvement in their ichthyosis. As a result of an abnormality of the keratin (the skin barrier) in ichthyosis, chemicals readily penetrate to the deeper layers of the skin and cause inflammation and soreness. This point has to be considered if the patient seeks advice about the type of work which would be suitable for him.

### *Treatment*

Until recently there was very little one could offer patients with ichthyosis. Recently it has been shown that topical urea will improve keratinisation in patients with certain (the commoner) types of ichthyosis. The mechanism of action of urea in these forms of ichthyosis is not fully understood but it may be related to keratin bonding. Usually 10 per cent urea in a cream base should be applied daily, particularly after bathing. Urea is not stable and the preparation will lose its effectiveness with time. There are, however, a number of proprietary urea preparations in which the urea has been made stable. Patients also derive benefit from bathing with a 10 per cent coal tar solution B.P. in emulsifying ointment B.P. instead of ordinary soap.

It is most important to tell the patients to wear gloves in winter and keep their skin temperature as high as possible by suitable clothing. If secondary eczematisation occurs this should be treated with topical steroids.

A point to remember in patients with ichthyosis is that there is often occlusion of the sweat ducts and, thus, their tolerance to heat and exercise is reduced and febrile episodes must be taken seriously, particularly if the ichthyosis is extensive.

### Neurofibromatosis (von Recklinghausen's disease)

This is a disorder affecting the skin and nervous system. The classical signs are light brown macular lesions, so-called 'café-au-lait' spots (Figures 23.4 and 23.5). There are usually several such lesions but occasionally there may only be a few.

Café-au-lait lesions may be present at birth and often precede the development of skin tumours by years. Occasionally they are the only features of the disorder in the skin. If skin tumours develop they usually do so around puberty. The tumours arise from the Schwann cells of the cutaneous nerves. These tumours may be few in number or very numerous. The growths are usually skin coloured and may vary in size from a few mm to a few cm. They may be small round elevations (Figure 23.6) or they may be pedunculated or present as raised, soft plaques (Figure 23.5). The tumours are usually painless but may be painful if situated over a pressure area.

Neurofibromatosis affecting the skin is essentially a cosmetic disability but of serious medical importance are the neurofibromata which may be found on the cranial nerves or in the spinal canal.

There is no treatment for this disorder but if a tumour is particularly large or causes pain it can be excised.

### Epiloia (Tuberous Sclerosis)

This is a disease characterised by lesions in the central

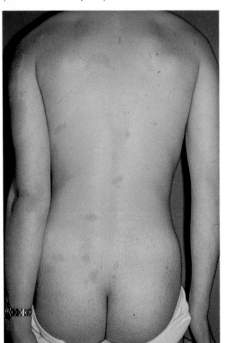

**Figure 23.4** *Pigmented, macular lesions ('café-au-lait' spots) in neurofibromatosis.*

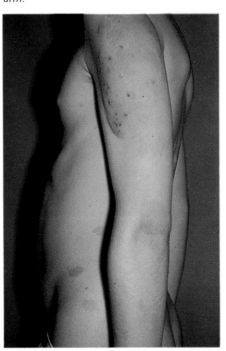

**Figure 23.5** *Café-au-lait patches and a large plaque neurofibroma on the upper arm.*

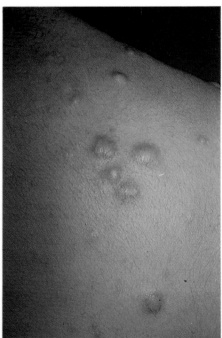

**Figure 23.6** *Nodular neurofibromata on the shoulder.*

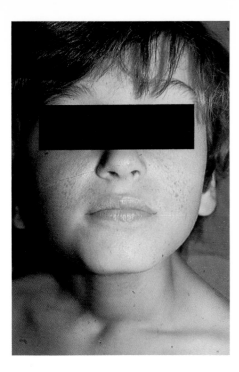

**Figure 23.7**
*Pink papules on the cheeks in epiloia.*

yellowish plaques usually situated in the lumbar region (Figure 23.8). They vary in size from 1 cm to 10 cm in diameter. The lesions are due to alterations in the dermal collagen. Occasionally there are fibrous outgrowths beneath the nails on the fingers and toes.

### Congenital Ectodermal Defect

This is a rare disorder and is due to failure of development of the skin and its appendages. There may be numerous abnormalities present or just one or two. The patients may present with bald patches in the scalp from birth due to absent hair follicles, the teeth may be absent, reduced in number and abnormally shaped. The sebaceous glands and sweat glands may not be formed. The clinical importance of this latter feature is intolerance to heat.

## Dermatitis Artefacta and Neurotic Excoriations

These are two disorders in which lesions are produced in the skin by the patient due to mental disease.

### Dermatitis Artefacta

In this disorder patients will never admit to producing the lesions whilst the physician is taking the history. The diagnosis is often arrived at for negative reasons because the skin lesions do not fit any clinical disease pattern, e.g. the symmetry of psoriasis or an endogenous eczema. The lesions themselves have features which suggest that they have been produced by some physical agent, e.g. chemicals, burns (usually from cigarettes) or trauma from a sharp instrument. There is usually ulceration or blister formation in the epidermis (Figures 23.9, 23.10 and 23.11). The lesions are discrete (Figures 23.9 and 23.10) and usually asymmetrical.

nervous system and skin. Anatomically, there are fibrous tumours in the brain while the presenting neurological features are mental deficiency and epilepsy. The skin lesions are characteristic and are not present at birth but usually appear during the first decade. The lesions are small pink papules situated in the naso-labial folds (Figure 23.7). They may spread to involve the cheeks below the eyes and the chin. The lesions have been termed 'adenoma sebaceum'. Other skin lesions in the disease are flesh coloured or

**Figure 23.9** *Discrete ulcers and scabbed lesions on the forearms in dermatitis artefacta. Scarring from previous lesions is present.*

**Figure 23.8** *Raised skin-coloured plaques on the back in epiloia.*

**Figure 23.10** *Discrete blisters and erosions in dermatitis artefacta.*

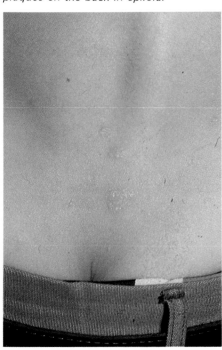

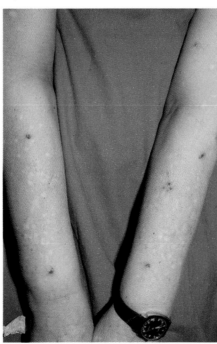

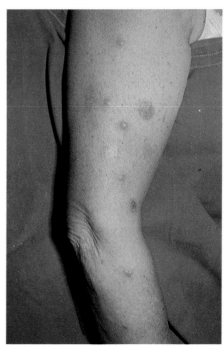

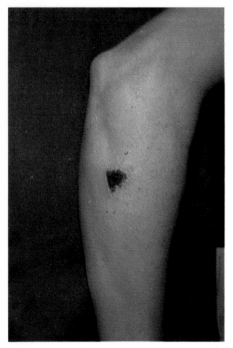

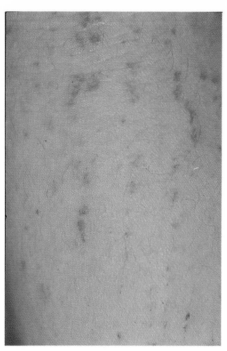

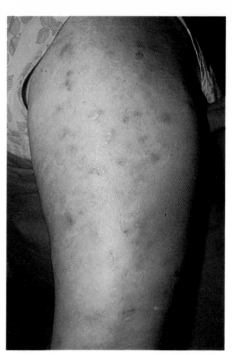

**Figure 23.11** *Deep, solitary, scabbed lesion in dermatitis artefacta.*

**Figure 23.12** *Neurotic excoriations. Linear superficial erosions due to scratching.*

**Figure 23.13** *Prurigo nodularis. Excoriated nodular lesions on the arm.*

The diagnosis of dermatitis artefacta is frequently missed at the first consultation and it is only when the lesions are failing to heal with conventional therapy and new lesions keep appearing, that the diagnosis is considered. To support the diagnosis it is sometimes necessary to apply occlusive bandages (in extreme cases plaster of Paris has been used) so that the patient can no longer inflict damage to the skin.

The disease is commoner in females than males at all ages. The patient usually has an hysterical personality and requires psychiatric treatment.

## Neurotic Excoriations

This is distinct from dermatitis artefacta because patients admit to scratching and the lesions are usually produced by the finger-nails, although some use mechanical aids.

The clinical presentation is that of linear superficial ulcers (Figure 23.12) although many will be in the healing stage and present as scabbed lesions. The lesions are usually found on the limbs and shoulders, the centre of the back is spared as the patient cannot reach this site. As in dermatitis artefacta the lesions will heal completely with occlusive dressings. However, these dressings only serve to confirm the diagnosis and the patient requires psychiatric treatment.

## Prurigo Nodularis

This is a distinct classical entity. It occurs most commonly in middle-aged females. The classical lesions are discrete, discoid excoriations, in which the skin becomes thickened and has a tendency to form nodules (Figure 23.13). The patients admit to excoriating the lesions as in neurotic excoriations, but the lesion produced is different. It is thought that the patients have an atopic tendency in which the skin becomes thickened due to trauma as with other forms of atopic eczema. The condition is persistent and resistant to most recognised forms of dermatological therapy. It is also resistant to psychiatric treatment.

# 24. Disorders of the Hair and Pigmentation

### Disorders of Hair

**T**HE common disorders of hair seen in a skin clinic fall into two categories—either loss of hair (alopecia) or excess hair (hirsuties). Hair loss can be classified into primary, where the fault lies in the hair or its production, or secondary, where the hair follicles are destroyed due to a disease affecting the dermis. Clinically, the latter type of alopecia is associated with scarring of the skin. To understand the basis of a number of pathological conditions it is necessary to have some knowledge of the 'hair cycle'. The hair growth cycle is divided into three stages—a growing phase (anagen) followed by a resting phase (telogen) during which the hair is shed and there is involution of the hair follicles, then finally, there is a stage of pronounced cellular activity of the hair follicle (catagen) prior to the actual production of the hair. There are approximately 100,000 hairs on the scalp and the normal daily loss varies from 20–100. This means that up to 100 hair follicles enter the telogen phase per day.

### Primary Hair Loss

From the clinical point of view it is often useful to consider hair loss as diffuse or patchy.

**Figure 24.1** *Male pattern baldness with hair loss over the vertex.*

### *Diffuse Hair Loss*

*Male pattern baldness.* Hair loss from the scalp in men is so common that it can hardly be considered to be abnormal. However, a number of young adult males do present to their own doctors and in skin clinics complaining of hair loss. There is a distinct pattern in this type of hair loss and it should be recognised so as to distinguish it from other causes of hair loss. Normal male pattern baldness begins in the temporo-frontal regions so that there is a receding frontal hair line at the sides. The next site to be affected is the vertex, particularly posteriorly extending on to the back of the scalp. If the hair loss is severe the only hair that remains is at the sides and lower part of the back of the scalp (Figures 24.1 and 24.2). It may begin in the late teens and once it commences it is usually progressive. However, the time over which this progressive hair loss occurs is extremely variable. Some patients lose all their hair on the vertex and frontal regions of the scalp in two to three years; others may gradually lose some of their hair but never become completely bald in the areas of the scalp involved.

There is no suitable therapy at the present time to reverse or stop male pattern baldness.

**Figure 24.2** *Male pattern baldness extends from the vertex to the back of the scalp. Hair is not lost from the sides or the lower part of the back of the scalp.*

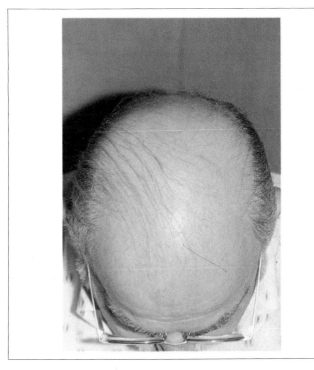

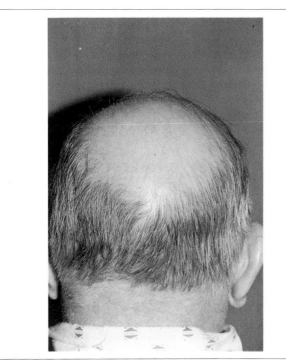

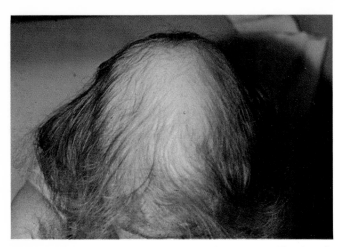

**Figure 24.3** *Constitutional hair loss in women. The loss is most marked from the vertex. The frontal hair line does not recede as in men and the hair loss is not total.*

*Hair loss in women.* So-called constitutional female alopecia is not an uncommon disorder seen in a skin clinic. It presents as a diffuse loss of hair from the scalp but the loss is mainly from the vertex. Although the hair loss may be severe it is not total as in men (Figure 24.3). The frontal hair line does not recede as in men. This type of hair loss is seen most commonly in middle-aged and elderly patients but it can occur in young adults. The cause for this type of hair loss is, as yet, unknown. However, occasionally there is underlying systemic disease which may give rise to hair loss which is indistinguishable from the so-called constitutional form. The two commonest disorders which may cause hair loss are hypothyroidism and iron deficiency anaemia, both readily treatable, so female patients complaining of gradual diffuse hair loss should be investigated to exclude these disorders.

Another cause of diffuse hair loss in females is traction on the hair resulting from certain types of hair styles. This is particularly so in negroes, including children, who plait their hair very tightly (Figure 24.4) or in women who sleep in 'hair rollers'. Thus inquiry should always be made concerning these habits. Unfortunately, there is no treatment for the constitutional type of hair loss in females. If it is very severe and the patient is distressed by her state then a wig should be advised. If severe traction is the cause of the hair loss then a change in hair style is all that is required.

*Telogen effluvium.* In this disorder a large number of hair follicles suddenly go into the resting phase of the hair cycle (telogen) and thus the hair is shed. The commonest causes for this type of hair loss are the 'post pregnancy state' and diseases often associated with high fever. It has also been reported after stopping the contraceptive pill. Although this type of hair loss may be severe (Figure 24.5) and very alarming to the patient, the condition subsides spontaneously after a few months and the hair cycle returns to normal. No treatment is available to stop the process but the patient should be strongly reassured as to the eventual outcome of the process and placebo therapy is sometimes helpful.

*Drugs.* A number of drugs may cause hair loss, the commonest being cytotoxic drugs. Hair loss has also been reported with heparin and excess vitamin A intake.

*Inflammatory dermatosis.* Hair loss does occur in some patients with seborrhoeic eczema and psoriasis but it is the exception rather than the rule. The cause of the hair loss is not known, but in some patients an aggravating factor is the trauma from continual scratching. In these conditions the hair loss is usually reversible.

**Figure 24.4** *Tight plaiting of the hair which may give rise to traction alopecia.*

**Figure 24.5** *Diffuse thinning of the hair in telogen effluvium.*

**Figure 24.6** *Oval bald patch on the scalp in alopecia areata.*

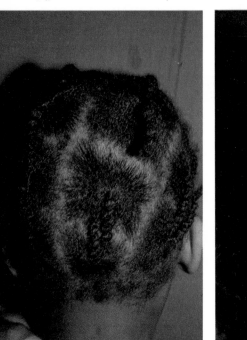

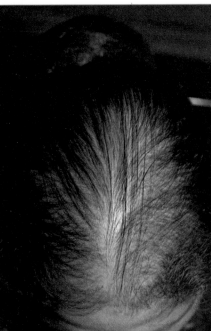

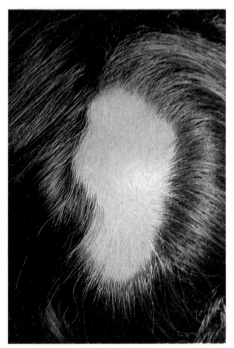

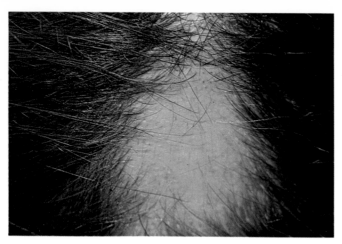

**Figure 24.7** *Exclamation mark hairs in alopecia areata. The hairs are short, 5 mm in length. They are thicker in their distal portions, the shaft tapering towards the proximal end.*

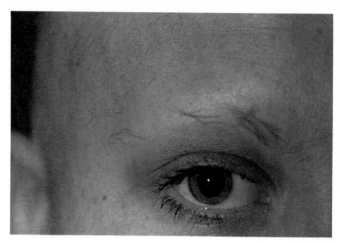

**Figure 24.8** *Alopecia areata involving the eyebrow.*

**Figure 24.9** *Alopecia areata of the beard area.*

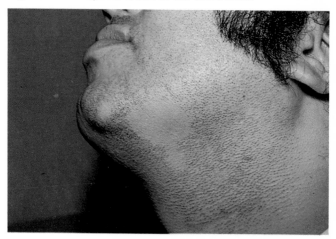

### Patchy Hair Loss

*Alopecia areata.* This is a relatively common disorder. The onset is fairly sudden, the patient noticing a round or oval bald area (Figure 24.6). The loss of hair may be complete or so-called 'exclamation mark hairs' may be seen in the bald patch or at the edges. Exclamation mark hairs are short hairs, approximately 5 mm in length, which are thicker at the distal part of the hair, the shaft gradually tapering towards the proximal end (Figure 24.7). If these hairs are pulled with forceps they come out very easily with a small white round lesion (the hair bulb) at the proximal end. Occasionally the scalp is slightly erythematous in the part affected. The skin itself is non-scaly (Figure 24.6) as opposed to the bald areas seen in fungus infection of the scalp. In alopecia areata there may be one or several bald patches. Occasionally, sites other than the scalp are involved e.g. eyebrows (Figure 24.8), or beard area (Figure 24.9). In rare instances, all the hair may be lost (Figure 24.10). This is termed alopecia universalis.

The most frequent course for alopecia areata to take is for the hair to regrow after an interval of time. However, time after which regrowth occurs is variable but is frequently two to three months. When regrowth does occur the hair is often white but usually repigments in time. Occasionally there is no regrowth of hair, whilst in other instances the hair regrows but new bald patches appear. Usually the larger the area initially affected, the worse the prognosis.

A feature sometimes seen in alopecia areata is dystrophy of the nails (Figure 24.11). This varies from a few pits to complete shedding. When dystrophy of the nails occurs, it is usually in the more severe cases of hair loss and is a poor prognostic sign.

*Treatment.* This is not very satisfactory. The only effective treatment is intralesional corticosteroids. The best way of getting the steroid into the dermis is by means of a dermojet (an instrument which injects fluid into the skin by means of pressure). The procedure is not painful whereas injection by syringe and needle into the scalp is. In severe forms of the

**Figure 24.10** *Total hair loss in alopecia areata. Hair is lost from all sites as well as the scalp—so-called alopecia universalis.*

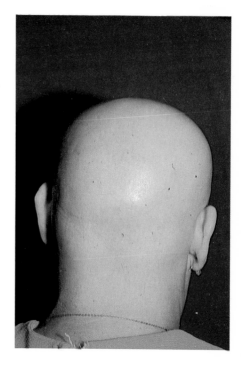

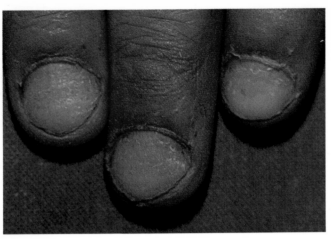

**Figure 24.11** *Nail dystrophy in alopecia areata.*

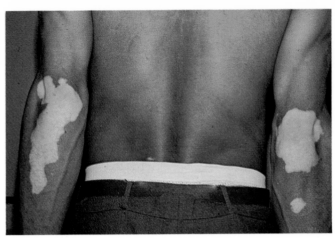

**Figure 24.14** *Symmetrical, oval, depigmented areas in vitiligo.*

**Figure 24.12** *Scarring alopecia secondary to an area of discoid lupus erythematosus.*

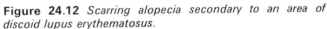
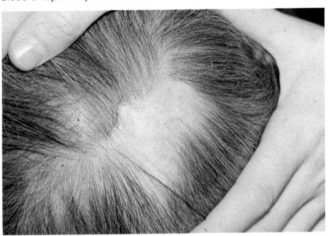

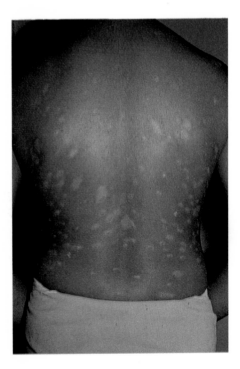

**Figure 24.13**
*Post-inflammatory hypopigmentation following psoriasis.*

disease the hair will regrow, where the steroids have been used, but after a few months the hair falls out again. If this happens then it is usually not worth continuing with the treatment and if the alopecia is extensive then a wig should be prescribed. Very occasionally it has been known for the hair to regrow spontaneously after many years of no growth.

Topical applications are of no use in alopecia areata and systemic steroids (although effective) should not be prescribed. There is regrowth of hair with systemic steroids, but if the disease is severe then the hair falls out again as soon as the steroids are stopped.

*Trichotillomania.* This is a disorder in which the patient has the habit of rubbing a particular area of the scalp or pulling the hair from a particular area. The disorder is commoner in children than adults. The presenting feature is a bald area but on close inspection it can be seen that the hairs have been broken close to the surface by trauma.

Most children grow out of the habit. If not, they should be referred to a psychiatrist.

*Congenital.* Bald areas occasionally occur from birth. This is due to failure of the skin to develop normally in these areas, the hair follicles being absent.

### Secondary Hair Loss—Scarring Alopecia

In any disorder in which there is severe inflammation of the dermis and subsequent scar tissue formed, the hair follicles will be destroyed with resulting baldness. This inflammation may be caused by burns, pyogenic infections or previous irradiation. These causes can usually be obtained from the history the patient gives.

A number of skin disorders, such as lichen planus, scleroderma and discoid lupus erythematosus may affect the scalp skin and produce scarring alopecia (Figure 24.12).

Scarring can usually be seen on examination of the scalp, the epidermis is frequently atrophic and the skin generally feels tight.

The only treatment that might be considered in some forms of scarring alopecia is plastic surgery but this would

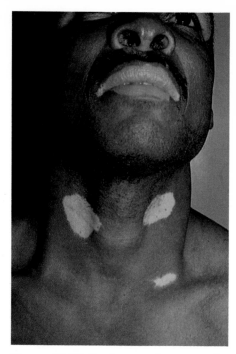

**Figure 24.15** *Depigmented areas on the neck in vitiligo. A severe cosmetic disability in a negro.*

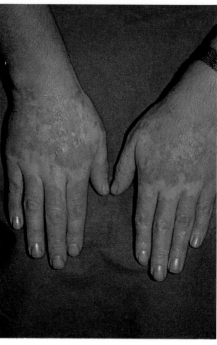

**Figure 24.16** *Symmetrical depigmented areas on the hands in vitiligo.*

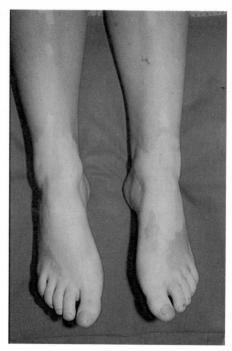

**Figure 24.17** *Large symmetrical, depigmented areas in vitiligo.*

only be applicable if the area involved was small and was due to a non-recurring cause, e.g. a burn.

### Hirsuties

Excessive hairiness may be localised or diffuse. In the vast majority of persons complaining of excessive hairiness there is no disease. Female patients present to doctors with this complaint because society does not accept excessive hairiness in women as normal, but it accepts it in men.

*Localised hirsutism.* This is most frequently found in association with benign pigmented naevi. Occasionally localised overgrowth of hair is found on the back, over the sacrum and lower lumbar spine.

*Essential hirsutism.* The amount of facial and body hair in women is in part genetically determined. Some facial hair and increased hair on the limbs is the norm rather than the exception in some Asians and in persons from the Southern Mediterranean countries. Excess hair growth in women may very occasionally be the presenting symptom of an endocrine tumour producing androgens. This is usually a tumour of the ovaries or adrenals. It must be stressed that this cause of hirsuties is extremely rare. As yet, the cause of essential hirsuties in women is unknown. No excess androgenic steroids or their precursors have been found in the serum but this could be due to the fact that the appropriate techniques have not yet been developed. Apart from excess production of the androgens in an endocrine gland there is now some evidence that the skin itself may be able to produce active androgens and thus the cause of hirsuties may be primarily a disorder of the skin itself.

When excess hair growth occurs in women it is found in similar sites to where body hair growth occurs in men, namely upper lip, beard area, lower abdomen from the pubis to the umbilicus and around the areolae on the breasts.

*Treatment.* It is important not to miss an endocrine abnormality as the cause of hirsuties in women. However, if the menstrual cycle is normal it is unlikely there is any under-

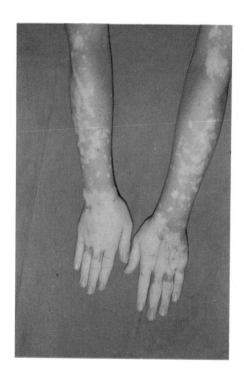

**Figure 24.18** *Extensive involvement in vitiligo.*

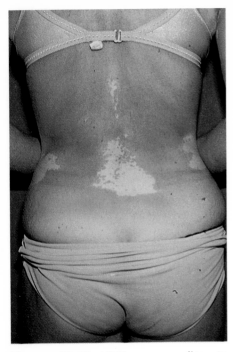

**Figure 24.19** *Vitiligo responding to treatment. Repigmentation occurs as small pigmented 'spots' in the affected area.*

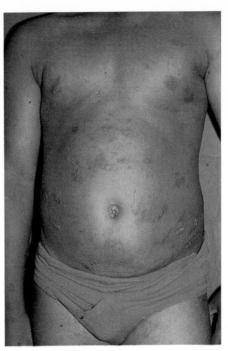

**Figure 24.20** *Post-inflammatory hyper-pigmentation secondary to eczema in a negro.*

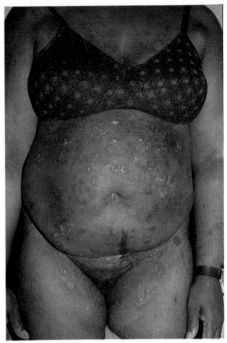

**Figure 24.21** *Post-inflammatory hyper-pigmentation associated with widespread fungal infection in a negro. The pigmentation is frequently the presenting symptom.*

lying tumour. Simple screening tests for tumours secreting androgens are not very reliable and the more sophisticated and reliable tests are time consuming and expensive and, therefore, should only be undertaken if the clinical state is strongly suggestive of a possible tumour.

The actual removal of the excess hair in essential hirsuties is not satisfactory. Temporary removal can be effected by plucking, depilatory creams, or, in severe cases, by shaving. The only permanent method of hair removal is by electrolysis. This is a time-consuming procedure and must be carried out by an experienced person to be effective. A number of endocrinologists have tried to treat hirsutism by oral corticosteroids and oestrogens to suppress the output by the adrenals and ovaries of hormones, some of which are androgens and, therefore, likely to cause excess hair growth. However, the results are not very good.

### Common Disorders of Pigmentation

#### Lack of Pigment

The commonest type of depigmentation of the skin seen in a skin clinic is post-inflammatory (Figure 24.13). The inflammation may have been due to any of the common skin disorders, e.g. eczema, psoriasis, pityriasis rosea. These depigmented areas usually become apparent once the dermatosis has cleared. One of the commonest sites for this phenomenon is the face in young children. If a careful history is taken there is usually a story of erythema and scaling preceding the eruption and frequently, on examination, scaling will be seen. Fortunately, the pigment returns after a few months and the only treatment required is that to suppress the primary inflammatory dermatosis.

#### Vitiligo

This is a distinct clinical entity. At the present time the cause is not known but there is increasing evidence that vitiligo is an immunological disorder which results in the inhibition of the formation of melanin by the melanocyte. There is a higher incidence of vitiligo in patients with 'auto-immune diseases', e.g. pernicious anaemia and some forms of thyroid and other endocrine diseases associated with auto-antibodies than in normal persons.

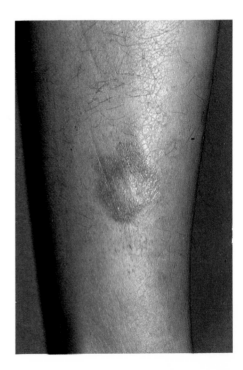

**Figure 24.22** *Post-inflammatory pigmentation after lichen planus.*

154

Vitiligo presents as oval or irregular white patches (Figures 24.14, 24.15 and 24.16). The lesions are frequently symmetrical (Figures 24.14, 24.16, 24.17 and 24.18). Occasionally there may be a solitary patch or sometimes the disease is very extensive involving large areas of the skin (Figures 24.17 and 24.18). Very rarely the whole of the skin may be affected.

The white patches of vitiligo are usually distinguished from other causes of depigmentation because the texture of the skin is normal. In some patients the hair becomes white in affected areas.

### Treatment

Vitiligo is a very embarrassing disorder for the patient if the depigmented areas are visible (Figures 24.15, 24.16 and 24.18). Although treatment is difficult and may fail it is certainly worth attempting if the patient feels particularly concerned about the appearance of his or her skin.

Two drugs are used in the treatment of vitiligo, corticosteroids and psoralens. Corticosteroids are used topically in a lotion or cream base. Only the potent topical corticosteroids appear to be effective in repigmenting the skin. Unfortunately the 'cure' rate with corticosteroids is low, no higher than 20 per cent. The treatment usually has to be continued for many months, and thus the patients have to be closely supervised because of possible side effects from the steroids. If there is no evidence of repigmentation within three months treatment should be discontinued. Vitiligo on the face is more likely to respond than that elsewhere.

The second drugs used in vitiligo are those of the psoralen group. Psoralens occur naturally in certain plants, but can also be synthesised. Psoralens have the ability, in the presence of ultra-violet light, to stimulate melanocytes to increase melanin production, and cause migration of melanocytes. Psoralens may be used topically or systemically. If there are only small areas of vitiligo then topical preparations should be used, but if the disease is extensive then the psoralen should be given by mouth, two hours prior to exposure to ultra-violet light. In suitable climates patients can use natural sunlight, but in temperate climates artificial sources of ultra-violet light are used. Long wave ultra-violet lamps are probably best, because these eliminate possible reactions due to short wave ultra-violet light. The initial exposure time is short, i.e. only a few minutes otherwise there may be severe phototoxic reactions. The supervision of vitiligo treatment is best undertaken by a specialist.

Negroes and Asians respond to treatment for vitiligo better than Caucasians. If repigmentation does occur, either due to psoralens or topical steroids, then it first appears as small 'spots' (Figure 24.19) in the white area. This is a useful sign for, if it does occur, it is a good prognostic sign and treatment should be continued. It is thought that the repigmentation occurs by melanocytes around the hair follicles migrating to the surrounding skin and then spreading across the depigmented areas.

If treatment with psoralens and topical steroids is not effective then the affected areas can be stained a 'brown

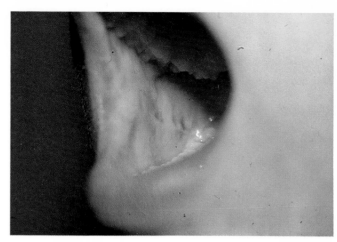

**Figure 24.23** *Buccal pigmentation. The buccal mucosa is a common site for areas of pigmentation in Addison's disease.*

**Figure 24.24** *Pigmentation on the lips in Addison's disease.*

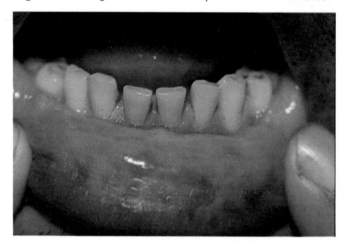

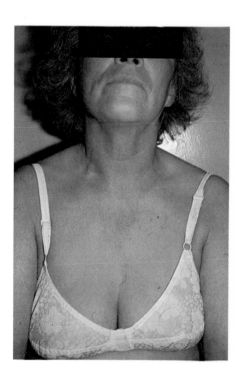

**Figure 24.25** *Generalised pigmentation in Addison's disease.*

155

colour' by the topical use of a number of substances. The one most commonly used is dihydroxyacetone.

## Increased Pigmentation

The commonest cause of increased pigmentation is post-inflammatory, usually following one of the common dermatoses (Figures 24.20 and 24.21) and particularly common after lichen planus (Figure 24.22). This well-documented phenomenon of post-inflammatory hyper-pigmentation is particularly common in negroes.

Patchy increased pigmentation may occur on the face and neck in women as a number of cosmetics are photosensitisers which increase the pigmentation of the skin following exposure to sunlight.

Increased pigmentation may be found in association with a number of systemic disorders e.g. Addison's disease (Figures 24.23, 24.24 and 24.25), malabsorption states, carcinomatosis, renal failure, Peutz-Jeghers syndrome, Albright's disease, haemachromatosis and neurofibro-matosis. These are disorders which belong to the realms of 'general' or 'internal' medicine and descriptions will be left to the appropriate texts, but the dermatologist must be aware that the altered pigmentation of the skin may be the presenting feature in these diseases.

## Chloasma

This is increased pigmentation, usually on the cheeks and forehead, which occurs during pregnancy (Figure 24.26) and in some patients taking the contraceptive pill. This type of pigmentation may also occur in females who are not

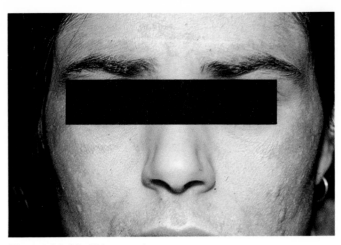

**Figure 24.26** *Chloasma in pregnancy.*

pregnant or taking the contraceptive pill, and is sometimes referred to as melasma. It is commoner in relatively dark skinned persons, particularly Asians, than in Caucasians. Chloasma after pregnancy in Caucasians usually fades spontaneously.

### Treatment

In simple post-inflammatory hyperpigmentation the colour of the skin usually returns to normal. If melanin hyperpigmentation persists, from whatever cause, the areas can be depigmented by the use of hydroquinones applied topically. They should be used with caution under the direction of a dermatologist.

# 25. Guides to Treatment

THE majority of medical students are never taught the basic pharmacological principles applicable to the treatment of skin disease. When he opens a book on skin diseases, even in this day and age, the student is confronted by a variety of ointments, creams, lotions, pastes, etc., many of which have been in use over the last 50 or more years and the great majority of which are useless in the management of most skin disorders.

The first decision to make in the treatment of a skin lesion is whether systemic or topical treatment is required. If the lesion is dermal as opposed to epidermal then topical measures will be of little or no use. Clinically, the lesion is dermal and not epidermal if there is no scaling, crusting, or weeping of the skin's surface. Topical measures are of no value in dermal disorders for two reasons. Firstly, if the epidermis is intact then it is unlikely that a high enough concentration of the drug will penetrate the skin barrier (normal keratin). Secondly, if the drug does penetrate the epidermis and reaches the dermis then it is absorbed into the tissue fluid and blood stream and is quickly diluted at the site where it is hoped that it will act. Conversely, if the lesion is mainly or partly epidermal, suggested on clinical grounds by scaling, crusting or weeping of the skin's surface, topical preparations are indicated. Topical preparations are likely to be more effective in this situation because the epidermal barrier has been destroyed by the disease process and, secondly, the epidermis has no blood vessels and so systemically administered drugs have to reach the epidermal cells by diffusion through the cells and intercellular fluid. Because of this a higher concentration of the drug can often be obtained in the epidermis by topical rather than systemic administration. The obvious advantage of the use of topically applied drugs as opposed to those systemically administered is that the diseased organ is specifically treated and the rest of the body is not exposed to the drug (or only in a very small concentration as compared to drugs given systemically).

## Vehicles for Topical Preparations

Students and practitioners are often confused because they have to know not only which drug should be used for the disorder but also in which vehicle the drug should be administered. Basically, topical preparations can be divided into four groups: solutions, creams, ointments and pastes.

**Figure 25.1** *Thinning of the skin due to prolonged use of topical steroids. Subcutaneous veins are easily visible.*

**Figure 25.2** *Thinning of the skin and purpura on the backs of the hands due to topical steroids.*

**Figure 25.3** *Extensive purpura on the forearm following long-term use of topical steroids.*

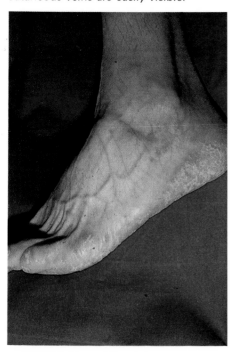
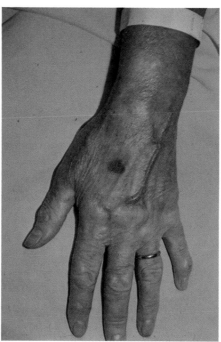
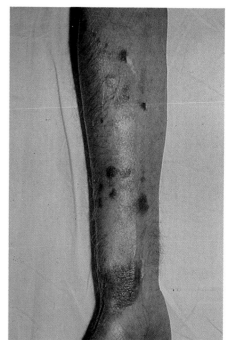

**Figure 25.4** (Right) *Striae in the groins and on the inner side of the thigh due to potent topical steroids in an intertriginous area.*

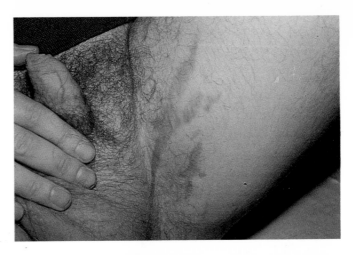

*Solutions.* The drug (e.g. steroid) should be used in solution form when the skin is acutely inflamed, as manifested by weeping or exudation from the skin's surface. Solutions are also indicated for dermatoses in the intertriginous areas (i.e. where two skin surfaces are in opposition, e.g. groins, axillae and between the toes). It should be appreciated that solutions will evaporate quickly if applied to the skin's surface and thus the duration of action of the drug on the diseased area is relatively short, perhaps only half an hour. Thus, if continuous treatment of the surface is required, lotions have to be applied frequently (e.g. hourly).

*Creams* are emulsions, either of water dispersed in oil, or of oil dispersed in water. They have a relatively high water content compared to the oil content. Clinically, this means they are pleasant and non-greasy to use and the patients will find they 'rub in' well. A cream should be chosen as the vehicle for the drug in subacute conditions, e.g. when there is slight exudation, and for disorders affecting the intertriginous areas. The duration of action of the drug can be expected to be longer than that of a solution but shorter than an ointment. It is probably of the order of 4 to 5 hours. Thus, if continuous treatment of the diseased skin is required the cream should be applied four to five-hourly.

*Ointments.* Clinically, these are substances which are 'greasy'. Chemically they may be of three different types: those which are water soluble, those which emulsify with water and those which do not mix with water. However, it is the clinical 'properties' which are important. Because these substances are greasy, they should not be used for acute weeping or subacute skin diseases or used in the intertriginous areas, particularly the groins and under the breasts. The main indication for their use is the presence of 'dry' chronic dermatoses. The duration of action of the drug in an ointment base is longer than that in a cream and thus it need only be applied two to three times a day for a continuous action of the drug on the skin. As a general rule, a drug (particularly a steroid) in an ointment base is more effective than the same drug in a cream base.

*Pastes.* These are ointments which have zinc oxide added to them, giving them a stiffer consistency. They are used only in chronic dermatoses, e.g. psoriasis. They will remain on the skin surface for a considerable length of time and need only be applied once a day. They are not pleasant for the patient to use.

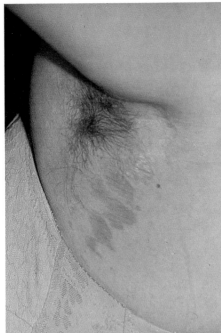

**Figure 25.5** *Striae in axilla, following long-term use of topical steroids.*

### Drugs

As far as treatment of skin disease is concerned, 99 per cent of conditions can be treated by approximately half a dozen drugs.

### Topically Applied Drugs

*Steroids.* At the present it would seem that the pendulum has

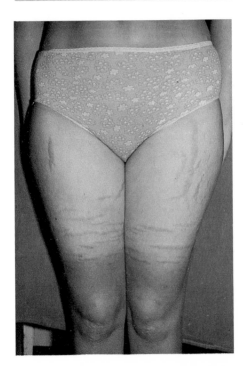

**Figure 25.6** *Striae in a non-intertriginous area, following long-term use of of potent topical steroids.*

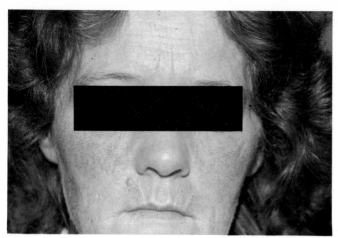

**Figure 25.7** *Telangiectasia on the cheeks after long-term topical steroids.*

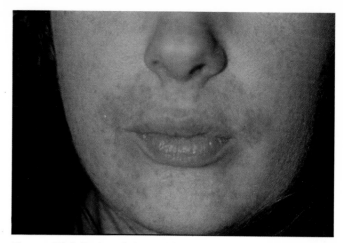

**Figure 25.8** *Peri-oral dermatitis.*

**Figure 25.9** *Spread of peri-oral dermatitis.*

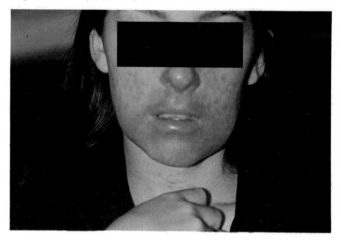

swung too far against topical steroids, particularly the potent members of this group, and a number of patients are being deprived of the benefits of these drugs. Topical steroids are potent anti-inflammatory preparations and are indicated in inflammatory disorders, particularly eczema. Bacterial and fungal infections should always be considered before prescribing or re-prescribing topical steroids, particularly if the dermatosis is not responding to treatment.

Patients using topical steroids on a long-term basis should not be given repeat prescriptions without the doctor examining the skin. At the end of this chapter a list of the commoner topical steroid preparations grouped in order of potency is given. Because there are now so many topical steroids available it would seem sensible to become familiar with one or two steroids from each group and stick to them. If large quantities of topical steroids are required for extensive and chronic skin disorders, it is considerably cheaper to dilute the stronger topical steroids with a suitable diluent than to prescribe the same quantity of a proprietary dilute steroid. If diluents are to be used then it is best to use one proprietary steroid and learn the appropriate diluent, as different proprietary topical steroid preparations require *different* diluents. The appropriate diluent can be obtained by consulting 'The External Diluent Directory' which is available to pharmacists or by contacting the pharmaceutical company which produces the steroid. The amount by which the proprietary steroid is diluted will depend on the strength required, but it is usually diluted four to five times. In clinical practice, now that very potent topical steroids are available, it may be wiser to use short courses of these potent drugs in the treatment of chronic eczemas and psoriasis to clear the condition (if only for a short while) rather than simply attempting to keep the condition to tolerable proportions by the continuous use of a weaker steroid.

### Adverse Effects of Topical Steroids

As a rule, the side effects of topical steroids are proportional to the product of strength of the steroid and the duration of use. However, it must be remembered that when these substances are used in areas where the skin is thin (e.g. the face) and in intertriginous areas where there is greater absorption of steroid into the skin due to moisture, the risk of side effects is greater.

*Topical side effects.* Steroids suppress formation of new collagen, and cause atrophy of collagen in the dermis. Clinically this may present as thinning of the skin, which will have a wrinkled appearance, and the subcutaneous veins become prominent (Figure 25.1). Purpura develops at sites of minor trauma, usually the backs of the hands (Figures 25.2 and 25.3) and legs. Striae (which are usually irriversible) are most likely to be seen in the moist intertriginous areas (Figures 25.4 and 25.5) due to greater absorption of steroid into the skin. However striae will also appear on non-intertriginous skin after prolonged use of steroids (Figure 25.6).

Prolonged use of potent topical steroids on the face will lead to thinning of the skin and telangiectasia (Figure 25.7). In some persons, particularly if the drug is used to treat seborrhoeic eczema, there is an idiosyncratic response to the drug. The patients develop a papular eruption around the mouth (Figure 25.8), and this eventually spreads to the cheeks (Figure 25.9), eyelids and even the forehead. When the steroid is discontinued there is a worsening of the condition, which has been termed circumoral or peri-oral

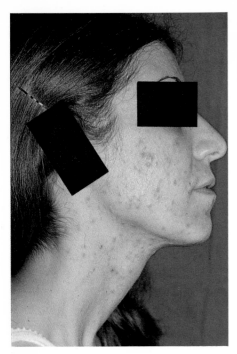

**Figure 25.10** *Acne induced by topical steroids.*

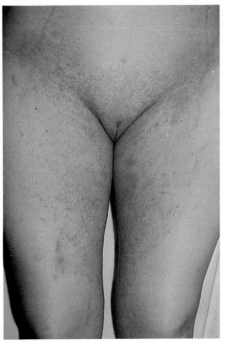

**Figure 25.11** *Fungal infection of the groins (which has spread to the thighs) treated with topical steroids for five years. Scaling and a definite edge are absent.*

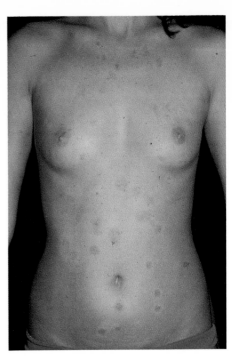

**Figure 25.12** *Fungal infection on the trunk treated with topical steroids; annular configuration is absent.*

dermatitis. Treatment of the condition is by gradual weaning of the patients from potent topical steroids to weak topical steroids and systemic tetracyclines. Potent topical steroids used on the face may also induce acne (Figure 25.10).

If topical steroids are used for fungal or bacterial infections they may mask the usual clinical presentation and lead to diagnostic difficulties. This is particularly so with fungal infections of the skin in which the scaling and annular configuration disappears (Figures 25.11 and 25.12). Viral infections, particularly herpes simplex infection, may spread if topical steroids are used in the management of the condition.

Care is needed when topical steroids are used for treatment of dermatoses on the eyelids. Increased ocular pressures have been reported as a result of topical steroid being absorbed through the conjunctiva into the eye.

*Systemic side effects.* Systemic side effects following the use of topical steroids are extremely rare. The side effects are proportional to the product of potency of the topical steroid and the quantity of steroid used. Thus the risk is greater when potent steroids are used over large areas of skin. The commonest side effect is suppression of the adrenal pituitary axis. There are a few reports of Cushing's disease and even diabetes mellitus having been precipitated by topical steroids.

*Topical antibiotics.* These can be combined with topical steroids or used alone. They are only effective in epidermal disorders, or when the epidermis has been destroyed. Remember that topical antibiotics are potential sensitisers.

*Topical antihistamines and topical local anaesthetic preparations* have no part to play in the treatment of skin disease. They are potential sensitisers and topical steroids are more effective in controlling inflammation and irritation associated with epidermal disorders.

*Tar preparations* still have a definite part to play in the management of some patients with psoriasis. They may occasionally be helpful in persistent eczematous lesions. In psoriasis, crude coal tar is usually used at a concentration of 5 per cent in an ointment base (soft paraffin) or a paste (Lassar's paste). Fifteen per cent coal tar solution in emulsifying ointment B.P. is helpful in the treatment of chronic eczematous lesions. It should be applied in liberal quantities to the trunk and limbs prior to bathing and the use of soap should be avoided. When this preparation is used the patient should stay in the bath for fifteen minutes and use the ointment as a soap substitute as it has some cleansing properties.

*Potassium permanganate soaks.* At a dilution of 1:8000 potassium permanganate solution is effective in helping to control acute inflammatory dermatoses, e.g. weeping or blistering eczematous lesions or fungal infections.

*Magenta paint.* This is a relatively 'old fashioned' remedy but it is often helpful in controlling a dermatosis affecting an intertriginous area. It has mild antifungal, antibacterial and antimonilial properties.

*Topical antifungal preparations.* Learn one and stick to it. Whitfield's ointment (benzoic acid co. oint. B.P.C.) still appears to be as effective as many of the newer preparations.

Probably its only indications are fungal infections of the feet and, after it has been diluted to half strength, pityriasis versicolor.

*Nystatin* is specific for monilial infections. It is usually combined with a topical steroid preparation. Nystatin is not effective against ringworm fungi.

## Systemic Drugs

*Griseofulvin.* This is an antifungal antibiotic. It has to be given systemically and has no effect in pityriasis versicolor or against monilia. In the treatment of fungal infections of the skin it has to be given for four weeks, for infections of the scalp six weeks, and for the finger nails for six months. For infections of the toe nails its value is questionable.

*Antibiotics.* Apart from their use to treat skin infections, antibiotics are used extensively in the treatment of acne. The tetracyclines are still the commonest drugs used for this purpose, and they are also used in the management of rosacea and peri-oral dermatitis.

*Antihistamines.* These drugs have an antipruritic action. Many of them make patients drowsy, which is useful at night but not during the day. Their main indications are in the control of pruritus and in the treatment of urticaria.

*Steroids.* The main point concerning systemic steroids in the treatment of skin disease is that the indications for the use of these drugs are very few and should best be left to a dermatologist.

# Appendix 1

## NAMES OF DRUGS

| | Generic Name | Trade Name UK | Trade Name US |
|---|---|---|---|
| **Topical Steroids** | | | |
| **Very Strong** | Clobetasol propionate (0.05%) | Dermovate | |
| | Fluocinolone acetonide (0.2%) | Synalar Forte | Synalar HP |
| | Beclomethasone dipropionate (0.5%) | Propaderm Forte | |
| **Strong** | Betamethasone valerate (0.1%) | Betnovate | |
| | Betamethasone (0.2%) | | Celestone |
| | Fluocinolone acetonide (0.025%) | Synalar | Synalar |
| | | | Fluonid |
| | Halcinonide (0.1%) | Halciderm | Halog |
| | Fluocinonide (0.05%) | Metosyn | Lidex |
| | Beclomethasone dipropionate (0.025%) | Propaderm | |
| | Fluclorolone acetonide (0.025%) | Topilar | |
| | Triamcinolone acetonide (0.1%) | Adcortyl | Aristocort |
| | | Ledercort | |
| | Fluocortolone pivalate (0.25%) + fluocortolone hexanoate (0.25%) | Ultralanum Plain | |
| | Fluocortolone (0.25%) + fluocortolone hexanoate (0.25%) | Ficoid 5 | |
| | Flumethasone pivalate (0.02%) | Locorten-Vioform | |
| | Flumethasone pivalate (0.03%) | | Locorten |
| **Intermediate Strength** | Clobetasone butyrate (0.05%) | Molivate | |
| | Hydrocortisone butyrate (0.1%) | Locoid | |
| | Flurandrenolone (0.0125%) | Haelan | |
| | Flurandrenolone acetonide (0.025%) | | Cordran |
| | Fluocortolone pivalate (0.1%) + fluocortolone hexanoate (0.1%) | Ultradil | |
| **Weak** | Hydrocortisone (0.5%, 1% and 2.5%) | Efcortelan | Cort-Dome |
| | | Hydrocortistab | Cortril |
| | | Hydrocortisyl | Dermacort |
| | | Hydrocortone | Heb-Cort |
| | | | Hytone |
| **Some Useful Topical Antibiotics** | Sodium fusidate (2.0%) | Fucidin | |
| | Gentamicin (0.3%) | Cidomycin | |
| | | Genticin | |
| | Gentamicin (0.1%) | | Garamycin |
| | Neomycin sulphate (0.5%) + zinc bacitracin (500 units per g) | Neobacrin | |
| | Neomycin sulphate (0.25%) + gramicidin (0.025%) | Graneodin | |
| | Neomycin sulphate (0.5%) | | Myciguent |
| **Some Anti-fungal Preparations: Against Ringworm Fungi** | Whitfield's ointment (benzoic acid 6%, salicylic acid 3%, emulsifying ointment 91%) | | |
| | Clotrimazole (1%) | Canesten | Lotrimin |
| | Miconazole nitrate (2%) | Dermonistat | Micatin |
| **Against Candida Albicans:** | Nystatin (100,000 units per g) | Nystan | Mycostatin |
| | | | Nilstat |
| | Amphotericin (3%) | Fungilin | Fungizone |
| | Clotrimazole (1%) | Canesten | Lotrimin |
| | Miconazole nitrate (2%) | Dermonistat | Micatin |
| **Useful Sun Screen: Against short wave ultra-violet light (290–320 nm)** | Isoamyl–p–N N–dimethylamino-benzoate (2.5%) | | |
| | Octyl dimethyl PABA (3.3%) | Spectraban | Sundown |

# Index